30 DAYS
to SUPER ABS

TRIM & TIGHTER AT ANY AGE, ANY BODY SHAPE

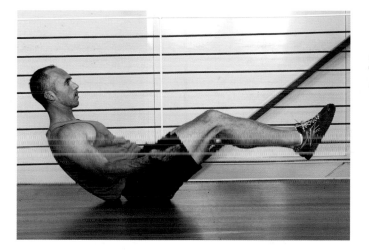

Damien Kelly

Published by:
Wilkinson Publishing Pty Ltd
ACN 006 042 173
Level 4, 2 Collins St Melbourne, Victoria,
Australia 3000
Ph: +61 3 9654 5446
www.wilkinsonpublishing.com

International distribution by Pineapple
Media Limited (www.pineapple-media.com)
ISSN Number: 2203-2789

National Library of Australia Cataloguing-in-
             Publication entry
Creator: Kelly, Damien, author.
Title: 30 Days to Super Abs / Damien
             Kelly.
ISBN: 9781925265125 (paperback)
Subjects: Abdominal exercises - Physical
fitness - Exercise.
Dewey Number: 613.71886

The information within these pages is
intended as an educational resource only.
Any physical training you undertake, as a
result of reading this book or otherwise, is at
your own risk.

Photos by agreement with international
agencies and photographers including
Rodney Stewart, Dreamstime and Getty
Images.

Design: Melinda Ayre
Printed in China.

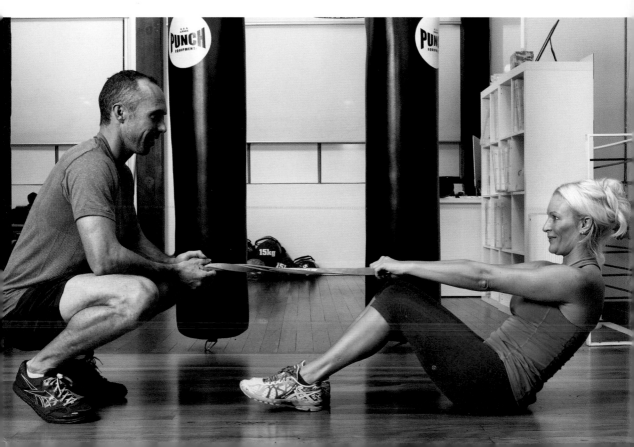

contents

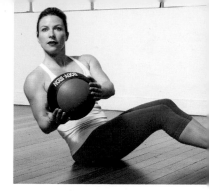

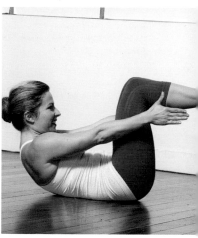

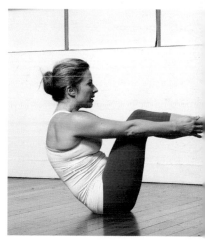

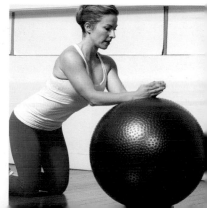

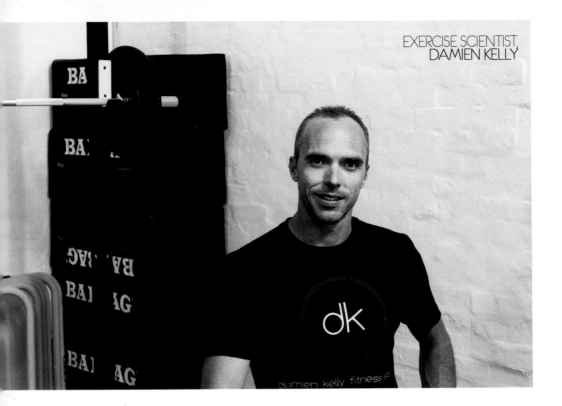

about damien

Damien Kelly is a qualified Exercise Scientist with over seventeen years experience in the fitness industry as both a professional trainer and fitness journalist. Damien is highly regarded within the industry for his unique, meticulously planned whole body programs.

Damien's workouts and no-nonsense, science-based fitness advice were featured in the *body+soul* lift-out in News Limited publications for over 10 years and read by millions of Australians weekly.

Currently, Damien runs two Sydney-based fitness studios, which showcase his small group training system based on bespoke, circuit-style workouts delivered in a highly supervised environment.

He lives with his partner Melinda and their two children, Finley and Venus.

foreword

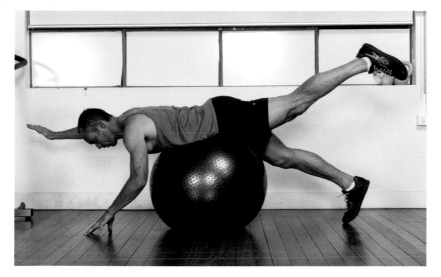

30 days to super abs...

If you've read my previous books or blogs and know anything about my style of training, you'll know I'm a huge fan of whole-body training. I rarely encourage my clients or followers to isolate one part of their body. So why am I blatantly breaking this rule and writing a book solely on training the muscles in your torso?

Well these muscles are special on two fronts. Firstly, they're integral to everything we do physically and form the basis for all other movement. There is not one exercise that doesn't involve these muscles. Secondly, almost nobody is doing these exercises correctly and therefore are not able to garner the intended benefits. Abs and core training needs a thoughtful and direct approach. These muscles are difficult to engage and your body will always take the easier way out. For effective abs training, insider knowledge is crucial and therefore I believe the abs deserve a book all their own.

It's my intention that after reading this book and completing the 30 day challenge, you'll be an expert in all things abs and core. You'll know what it takes to get this troublesome area of your body trim, taut and terrific and you'll know how to properly activate these tricky, often lazy muscles.

The challenges in this book will launch you into a lifetime of super effective and enjoyable training. Training that will have you not only ripped (if that's your wish) but moving through life with good posture and without back pain. How wonderful to have a body you can trust to move how you desire and allow you to do the things you want.

Enjoy the read and the challenge!

Damien Kelly, Exercise Scientist

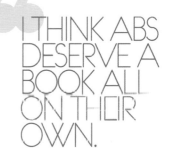

I THINK ABS DESERVE A BOOK ALL ON THEIR OWN.

how to use
this book

This book has two intertwined parts. Part one, which I'm sure you're most excited about, is the 30 Days of Abs Challenge. A top abs and core move every single day for 30 days to get your abs lean and toned. The second part of this book has loads of expert information to help you get the most out of these 30 exercises. You'll gain an understanding of the difference between abs and core as well as insider tricks to help you approach your abs training in the best possible way. I've pieced together all my fitness knowledge and experience from years of training my clients. Don't feel you need to read all the tips before you start the exercises. Read a couple, implement the key messages, and then move through the tips over the 30 day program.

is this book for me?

Yes - all of us can benefit from good abs and core training. Man or woman, young or old, fit or unfit, there is a lot in this book for you. Our abs and core are the hardest part of our body to train. They're made up of lazy muscles that are hard to engage. They often get left out of programs and shoved into the too-hard basket. I'll teach you all the little tricks to becoming an abs master. I'll challenge you to do better and help you tailor the challenges to your individual needs. All you have to do is get started on day one, make a 30-day commitment to see it all the way through and reap the rewards.

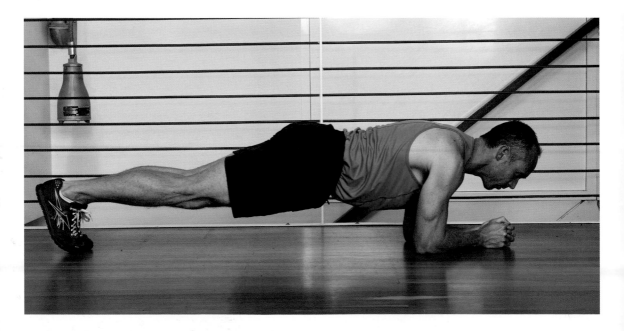

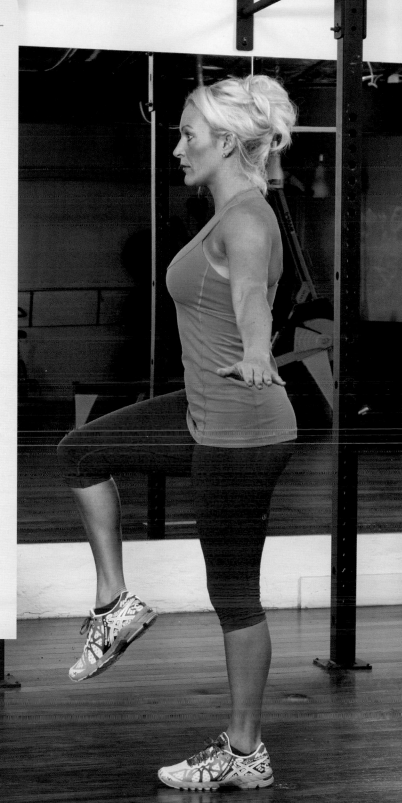

the levels

On each day of the 30 Day of Abs Challenge there are three different targets. Each daily challenge can be performed in one sitting or in bite size chunks through the day.

red level - beginners

The RED target is designed to be the most achievable and suitable for those just starting out on their fitness journey or those returning to training after time off.

blue level - intermediate

The BLUE target is a great target for those who've been training regularly for a while and are fairly proficient at the exercises.

black level - advanced

The BLACK target is programmed to be a real challenge, yet certainly attainable for experienced fitness buffs.

Don't feel like you need to stick to the same colour each day. On a day where you have plenty of time and find the exercise manageable, you may want to strive for the black level. The next day you may be flat out at work and find the exercises difficult so you may do blue.

scoring

To use for future reference, I'd like you to score each day. You get 0 points if you don't achieve the RED target, you get 1 point if you do. You get 2 points if you achieve the BLUE target and 3 points if you make it all the way to the BLACK target. Record your score each day in your book on the relevant page then add them together at the end of the challenge. NOTE: If targets like this intimidate you or are likely to demoralise you, just go through the program doing your best each day and be 100% happy with that.

YOUR TARGETS

Here's your targets for cumulative points for the entire 30 days:

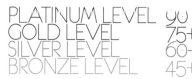

PLATINUM LEVEL	90
GOLD LEVEL	75+
SILVER LEVEL	60+
BRONZE LEVEL	45+

a new way to eat

Lean and clean eating for a trim tum is only a few small changes away, says food coach Jasmine Sakr.

If you want to get the most out of this fantastic 30 day abs program, your commitment towards better nutrition is paramount. Let's start by shutting off all the confusion about dieting and food fads. Together, let's start to create a new and improved mindset towards food. It's really quite simple: every time you eat, go for nutritional value. Intuitively select real, whole and traditional foods that will nourish and satisfy your body. *Change your food attitude* from 'this won't be so bad for me' to 'why is this good for me?'.

make small steps

Don't expect that you can get the body of your dreams overnight - true health is an evolving journey you'll be travelling your whole life. Unrealistic pressures often end in failure, so set yourself achievable, weekly goals. Start with something simple like, 'I will eat green vegetables with my dinner every night this week' or 'I will start every day with a glass of water'. Slowly but surely, you will overhaul your nutrition and most importantly, create long-term, positive habits.

know your macronutrients

To get complete nutrition every meal and snack, choose quality carbohydrates, a smart protein and a small amount of sensible fat. Did you know carbs are generally classified as foods that 'grow in the ground' (fruits, vegetables and grains) while protein-rich foods 'walk and swim around' (meat, fish, eggs, dairy but also beans, legumes and soy)? Some examples of sensible fats essential for optimum health and weight management are extra virgin olive oil, avocado and oily fish. Avoid tricking your body into 'low calorie/ low fat/low carb' mock products - you will just end up with constant cravings.

focus on what you CAN have

Many people believe to trim their waistline, they have to constantly deprive themselves of certain foods, usually during yoyo dieting. This is a negative attitude that spells disaster. For successful weight loss, move the focus away from deprivation and towards introducing new, fresh and healthy foods into the diet. Change your mindset from feeling deprived to feeling fuelled. Shift your focus from 'I want this but I can't have this' to 'I can have this but I don't want this' and watch how easily you control your cravings.

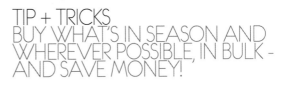

TIP + TRICKS
BUY WHAT'S IN SEASON AND WHEREVER POSSIBLE, IN BULK - AND SAVE MONEY!

it starts in your kitchen

Most healthy, lean folk prepare their meals themselves. Cooking doesn't have to be tiring or complicated. Instead, think of it as an important life skill, like driving a car. A delicious and nutritious meal is never far away if you stick to 4-5 ingredients (the recipes in this book are a good starting point). By committing to this program, you also agree to 'take out the garbage'. That means doing a thorough fridge and pantry clean and ridding your kitchen of processed, toxic products. Use your intuition and if you convince yourself into keeping those chocolate biscuits for an occasional treat, well, the only person you'll be failing is yourself. Once you've completed this important step, you're ready to sharpen your knives and fill your kitchen with fresh produce and quality cooking ingredients.

Cook

FOOD COACH,
JASMINE SAKR

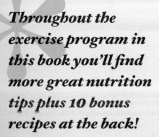

Throughout the exercise program in this book you'll find more great nutrition tips plus 10 bonus recipes at the back!

supermans

MOVEMENT TYPE
BRACE/TWIST

targets

	BLACK	BLUE	RED
	50	40	30

why?

One of the major mistakes we all make with abs and core training is getting fancy too quickly. If you haven't mastered the basics you'll never properly benefit from the more advanced exercises. This move is brilliant in its simplicity. Can you effectively engage your core while you raise your arm and opposite leg? The proof of this will be whether you can maintain a steady torso throughout.

how?

Assume an all fours position on the ground, knees under hips and hands under shoulders. Have your head in neutral (i.e. not too low or craned up). Simultaneously raise your arm and opposite leg off the ground. Raise the arm until it's level with the rest of your body. Keeping your leg relatively straight, raise until it's level to the rest of your body. Pause for a few seconds, lower and repeat.

Get a friend to place a tennis ball on the small of your lower back as you do this move. If you can keep the ball from falling off, chances are you're nailing this move.

your record

DATE	4/-7			
level reached	25			

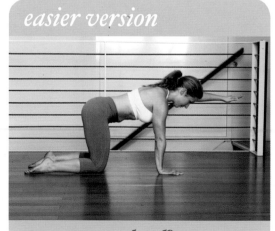

easier version

supermans too hard? Rather than raise your arms and legs simultaneously, simply raise one arm or one leg at a time.

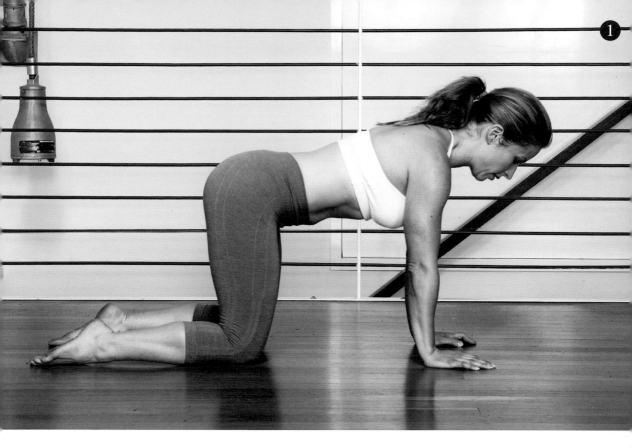

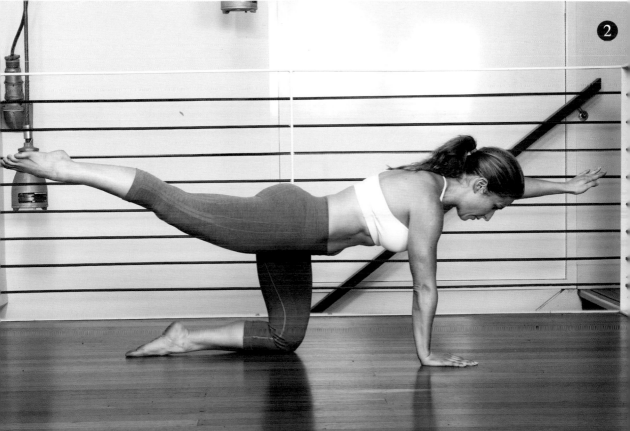

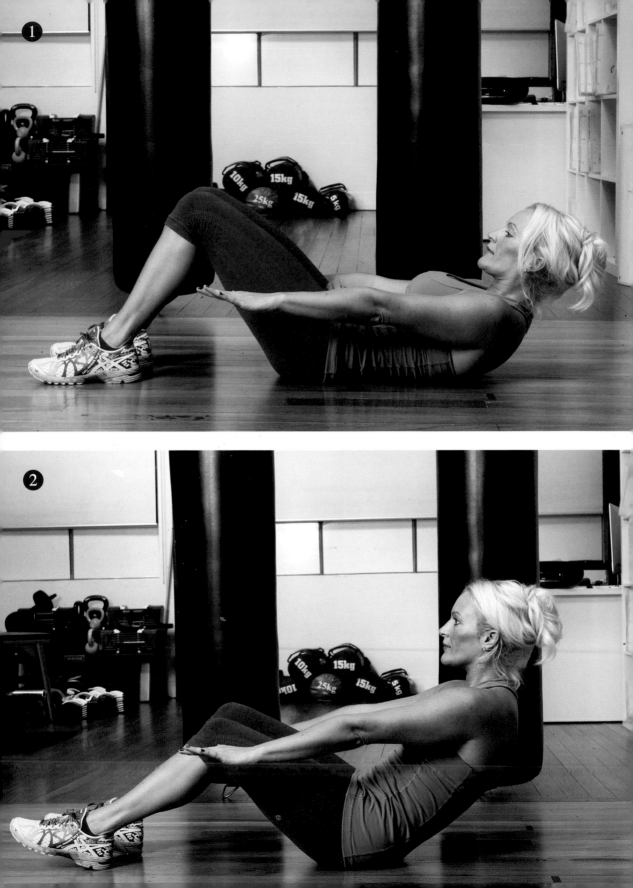

sit ups

**MOVEMENT TYPE
SPINAL FLEXION**

targets	BLACK	BLUE	RED
	100	70	40

why?

Over the years this has been the fitness industry go-to move when it comes to chasing the elusive six-pack. By itself it won't cut it, but nevertheless should play a part in the process.

how?

Lie on the ground with knees bent to 90 degrees, hands on thighs and head and shoulders raised off the ground. Squeeze and crunch your abs and sit up. Touch your ankles with your fingertips, then lower back to the ground. Lower until your shoulder blades touch then move straight back into your next rep. Be conscious of no jerky forward movements. Move slowly and at one consistent pace.

your record

DATE				
level reached				

> *Never hook your feet under an anchor while doing a sit up. This encourages the more dominant hip flexors to take over the movement leaving your abs unused. Aim to eventually do all your reps with feet anchored to the floor but not artificially.*

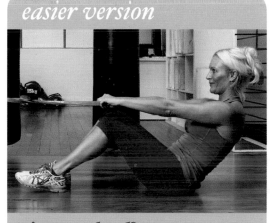

easier version

sit ups too hard? Sit near a post and wrap a skipping rope around it. Perform sit ups as normal but give yourself assistance (as little as you need) so you can move through the full range. Crunches won't help you get better at sit ups.

planks

MOVEMENT TYPE
BRACE

	BLACK	BLUE	RED
targets	10 min	6 min	3 min

why?

Like the sit up this is abs/core 101. And fair enough too. If, and I do mean if, done correctly it's a super simple and effective do-anywhere exercise that will firm your mid-section. I do however often see it performed incorrectly with hips sticking up in the air or lower back sagging.

how?

Lie flat on the ground. Go up into your usual push-up position but this time, rest on your elbows and forearms instead of on your hands. Look to a point just in front of your hands and grip your hands into fists. Engage your core muscles and lengthen your spine to fight downward sag. Breathe normally throughout.

Often you'll be thinking you're holding this position perfectly when you're not. Get a friend to watch or park yourself near a mirror so that you can ensure you're holding a straight, strong position.

your record

DATE	4/29			
level reached				

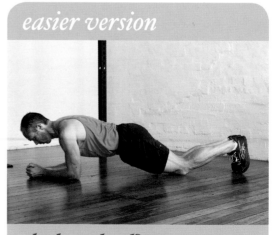

easier version

planks too hard? Try this either on your knees or alternatively with your forearms on a bench.

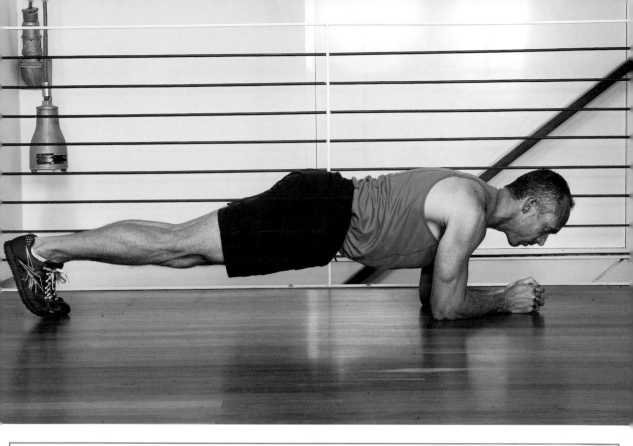

DID YOU KNOW? *Abs and core are not the same.*

In most of what you hear regarding training the area of your body between your ribs and hips, the words abs and core are loosely bandied between. But is this right? It's actually one of my pet hates when supposed experts do this because it shows a blatant misunderstanding for how this area of your body should be trained. Okay, so how do they differ from a training perspective?

core

A core exercise is any movement that challenges you to maintain posture. So whether it be gravity, movement or a weight (your body weight or external weight), if the movement is forcing your body to work to remain tall through the spine, it's a core movement.

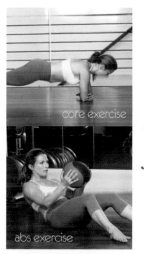

core exercise

abs exercise

abs

An abs exercise is where you actively leave posture. When I say actively I mean the purpose of the exercise is for your muscles to contract and flex the spine.

Every exercise will fall into one of these two categories. With the vast majority falling into the core category. If you do a core exercise and can't manage to maintain posture, it doesn't mean it's not a core movement, it just means you weren't able to meet the intended demand.

tips+tricks

1 *what is posture?*

When we talk about joints we often refer to their neutral position. This is the position in which they sit if they're healthy and no external force is acting upon them. Your spine is one long interconnected series of joints. Each vertebrae and disc working together to provide stability, strength and structure.

The neutral position of your spine, when considering the entire spine, takes the form of a soft 'S' shape. A flowing series of convex and concave curves. This genius design allows your body to do the things you require it to do. The spring-like series of curves giving you the ability to absorb the load and shock stemming from your movement.

Posture relates to when your spine is in a position of greatest strength and stability. Hunch or hyperextend and you are losing strength and becoming destabilised.

A handy way to ensure you're in fact in posture is to place your left index finger on your sternum and your right index finger on your belly button. While standing or sitting unsupported, lift these two points apart. You'll find your spine lengthen and your body straighten. Just ensure as you're doing this you aren't shrugging your shoulders.

2 *the tale of the apple core and the string*

Work your core daily and improve posture.

the apple core

> Stand tall and close your eyes (obviously you'll need to read this first!). Grasp the sides of your waist with your hands, thumbs at the back and fingers at the front, below your belly button but above your hip bones.

> Squeeze hands in from all sides to squish and decrease the size of your waist. Also strongly brace tummy muscles to draw waist in even more.

> While continuing to squeeze your muscles, release your hands. Your waist should still be greatly reduced. Next, reduce the intensity of your squeeze by half. Then by half again. And, yep, by half again. You should now feel a subtle brace, but you'll notice your posture is tall and tummy muscles firm.

> Now this is all well and good but what to do with this new party trick? Well, if you're doing a squat or deadlift (in laymans terms picking up a child or suitcase), perform this brace and hold it throughout the lift. The extra support will keep you safe and help you lift more weight, more often. Just be conscious that you don't force pressure down on your pelvic floor at the same time. Instead imagine you're pulling up through your pelvic floor as you brace. This will have the complete core musculature at its strongest.

the string

> The apple core is great when you're exercising but can't be maintained 24/7. That's where my second exercise comes into play. It requires the simplest bit of equipment of all time - a piece of string. Stand up tall and perform a light brace similar to you've just learnt. Pull up your shirt and get a friend to tie a piece of string around your waist at belly button level. This string acts as an alarm should you release your core muscles, as your stomach will expand and push out against the string. Ideally wear the string from the minute you wake until you again hit the sack. Wear it for a week straight so as to develop necessary core strength. Then do it once week as a core refresher after that.

3 *portion control*

MANY PEOPLE STRUGGLE WITH KNOWING WHEN TO STOP EATING. HERE ARE A FEW SIMPLE WAYS TO CONTROL PORTIONS:

> ENJOY AS MANY GREEN VEGETABLES AND OTHER FIBRE RICH FOODS AS YOU CAN, WHICH WILL MAKE YOU FEEL FULLER, FASTER.

> ENSURE EVERY MEAL AND SNACK IS A BALANCE OF SENSIBLE CARBOHYDRATES, PROTEIN AND FATS, WHICH WILL MAKE YOU FEEL FULLER, LONGER.

> EAT WHOLE FOODS AND WHOLE GRAINS INSTEAD OF WHITE REFINED FLOURS, BREAD, PASTA AND SUGAR.

> TREAT MEAL TIMES AS SACRED AND EAT MINDFULLY AWAY FROM ELECTRONICS AND TV. PAY ATTENTION TO THE MESSAGES YOUR BODY SENDS YOU ONCE YOU'RE FULL.

> USE SMALLER PLATES.

> SLOW DOWN AND CHEW EVERY MOUTHFUL FOR MAXIMUM NUTRIENT ABSORPTION AND METABOLISATION.

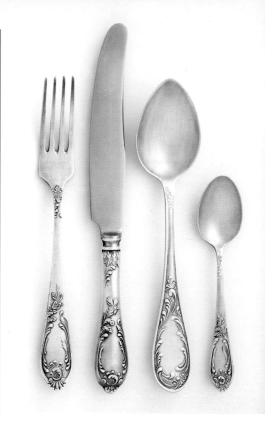

5 *eat for hunger (not boredom)*

IF THE PETROL TANK IN YOUR CAR WAS ALREADY FULL, WOULD YOU TAKE IT TO THE GAS STATION FOR A REFILL? RETHINK FOOD AS FUEL FOR YOUR BODY. THERE'S NO NEED TO REFILL YOUR ENERGY STORES UNLESS YOU MUST. BEFORE YOU REACH FOR SECONDS OR THAT SNACK AFTER DINNER, ASK YOURSELF 'AM I HUNGRY FOR THIS?'. IF NOT, THEN FIND OTHER WAYS TO ENJOY YOUR SPARE TIME, SUCH AS TAKING UP A NEW HOBBY OR RELAXING IN A HOT BATH.

4 *drink up*

Confusing thirst for hunger is one of the sneakiest tricks our body can play! Don't fall for it. Whenever hunger strikes between meal times, have a glass of water, then re-assess whether you're actually hungry. It may just be hydration you're craving. So how much water should you drink everyday? A good target is two litres, however individual needs change based on age, activity, climate, diet and health. Listen to your body and do what makes you feel best.

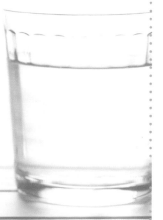

bump shifts

MOVEMENT TYPE
BRACE

		BLACK	BLUE	RED
targets		50	40	30

why?

I first saw this move for pregnant woman and while it's super effective for them it's also a super easy way for everyone to strengthen the side stabilising muscles.

how?

Lie on your side with your legs straight. Prop yourself up on your forearm by placing your elbow directly under your shoulder and have your forearm pointing forward. Raise your hips up off the ground and brace your tummy by imagining you're tightening a belt around your waist. Keep your neck in a neutral position. Hold for a second then lower your hip back to the ground. Almost touch then raise again. NOTE: You need to do today's prescribed reps on both sides.

your record

DATE	4/30			
level reached				

It's common when you get tired doing this move to lose your straight body position. Ensure throughout that your head is neutral, your hips are forward and your top shoulder doesn't fall forward.

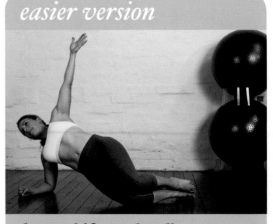

easier version

bump shifts too hard? Bend your knees to 90 degrees and rest on your knees, not your feet. Keep straight body alignment between your shoulders and knees.

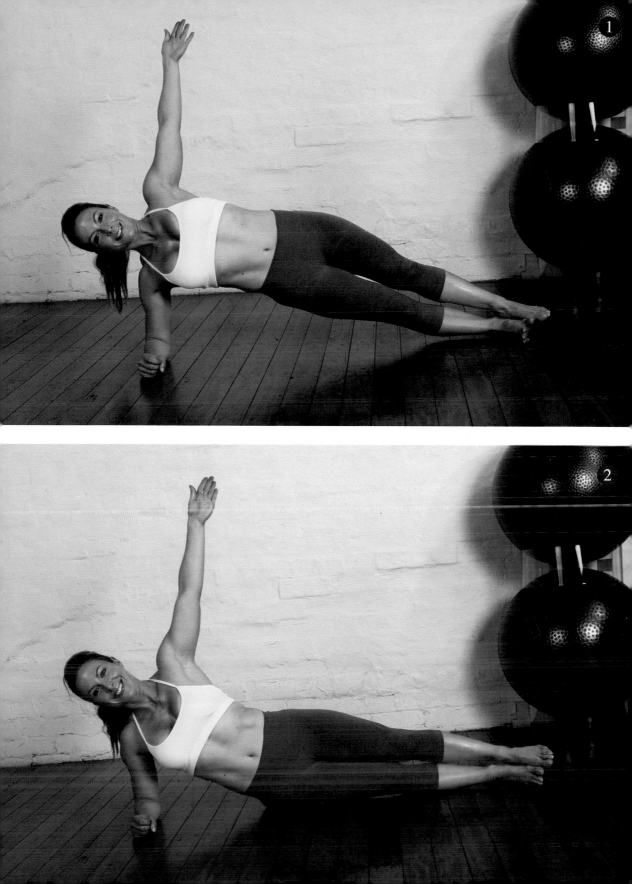

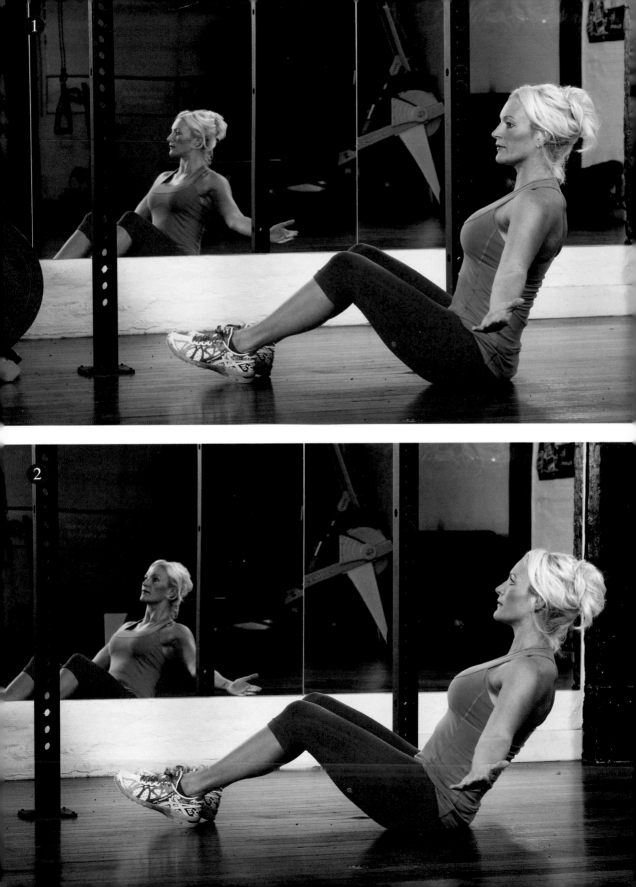

day 5

breaths

targets	BLACK	BLUE	RED
	50	40	30

why?

When programming, one of my considerations is varying the position your body is in. On day three I had you working your core muscles in a prone (face down) position. On day four I had you in a side lying position. Today we're simply mixing things up by performing another core focussed move but this time in a supine (face up) position.

your record

DATE				
level reached				

how?

Sit on the floor. Sit tall by lengthening the gap between your belly button and sternum. Maintaining this perfect posture, lean back with your torso 10-20 degrees. You will feel some shaking and shuddering in this position but hold steady for a series of three strong inhales and exhales. After the third breath sit back up to upright, that's one rep.

Be conscious to keep your head and neck in neutral by imagining you have an apple squeezed between your chin and chest.

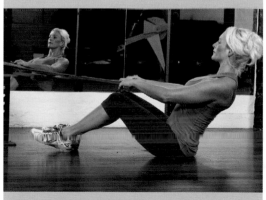

easier version

breaths too hard? In essence this is exactly the same exercise as the main version but the band makes you a bit lighter. This means a slightly easier time for your core. Ensure you don't round your upper back as you hold on and that you only hold on as little as you need.

day 6

cobra

MOVEMENT TYPE
EXTENSION

	BLACK	BLUE	RED
targets	50	40	30

why?

Sitting at your desk, in the car or in front of the TV has you in the unnatural position of triple flexion where the spine, hips and knees are all in simultaneous flexion. This in particular plays havoc with the health of our discs. The cobra is a genius move to counter this chronic flexion and helps to bring back nutrients and shape to our discs.

how?

Lie on your stomach on the ground and place your hands, palms down, underneath your shoulders. Be conscious to release any tension in your back and backside. Keeping your hip bones on the ground, press up safely, arching through your back. Try to ensure it's your arm strength doing the lifting and not your back or glutes. Try to get your arms as straight as possible but stop at the first sign of any lower back discomfort.

Although I have set you a reps target for today, I'd highly recommend you do the cobra on a daily basis. Ten reps twice a day may be enough to preserve the health of your spine for years to come.

your record

DATE				
level reached				

easier version

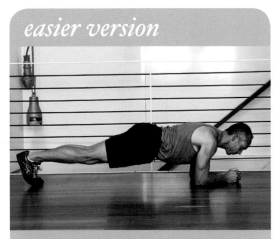

cobra too hard? If you do feel back pain as you do this or have a history of lower back disc issues, check with your doctor or physio as to the suitability and safety of this move for you. Alternatively, repeat the bridge today as your Day Six challenge.

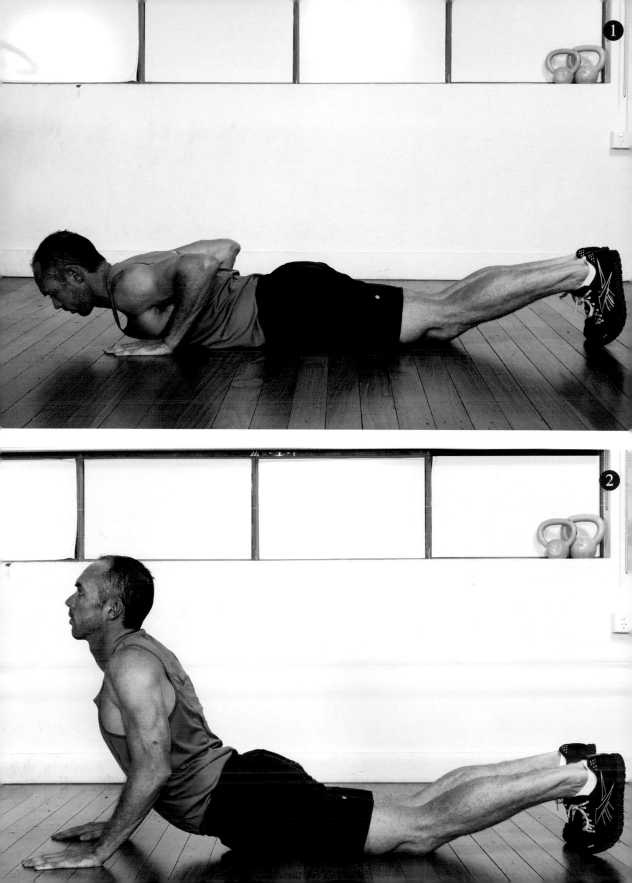

4 components of abdominal training

For most people the trusty old sit up is their go-to move when it comes to abdominal training, but if you've read my previous tips you may be starting to gather this won't cover it. In fact, a sit up only covers one of four important functions of our abdominal core area. Each of these four functions should receive as much attention as the others when it comes to your training.

You'll notice there is an equal sprinkling of each in my 30 day challenge and therein lies the key. Treat each with equal importance and you'll have the most balanced, sexy and ripped abs on the block. Here is a detailed breakdown of each component.

01 brace

WHAT IS IT?
Arguably the most important component. Bracing is your body's way of maintaining posture, against the external forces that life imposes on you.

WHAT DOES IT TARGET?
The TVA (transverse abdominis), which acts like a corset, runs belt-like around your mid-section between belly button and pelvis. A strong TVA means a safer back and slimmer tummy. Obliques are also important in bracing along with your pelvic floor and diaphragm.

WHAT SHOULD IT FEEL LIKE?
Not much really. It's more a sense than a burning sensation. You should feel firm as these muscles engage and feel a strength to your posture.

CAUTION?
There's danger of pressure on the pelvic floor, of particular concern for new mums. Learn the art of switching on and drawing up your pelvic floor as you brace - otherwise you can cause damage.

MUST KNOW?
Aesthetically, if your bracing muscles are weak or lazy and not engaged, your corset will relax and your lower tummy will stick out.

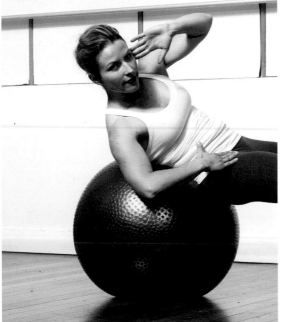

twist

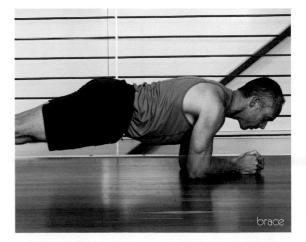

brace

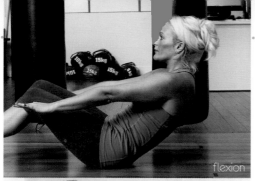

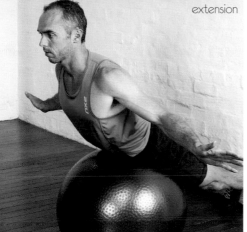

flexion

extension

03 flexion

WHAT IS IT?
Where you crunch forward and shorten the gap between your lower ribs and pelvis.
WHAT DOES IT TARGET?
This isolates the six-pack muscles (officially called the Rectus Abdominis)
WHAT SHOULD IT FEEL LIKE?
These muscles are very sensitive. If they're working they'll squeal loudly. By squealing I mean burning. The stronger the burn, and I'm talking eye-watering, the more effective your technique.
CAUTION?
The six-pack muscles are lazy and notoriously hard to target properly. Add to this the issue of the hip flexor muscles that live close by. This group of muscles are some of the most overactive in our body and if you're
not careful will dominate any intended six-pack move.
MUST KNOW?
Never hook your feet under an anchor when doing moves like sit ups and crunches. This will make it almost impossible to get an effective abs workout.

02 twist

WHAT IS IT?
Twisting through your mid-section.
WHAT DOES IT TARGET?
Predominantly your obliques
WHAT SHOULD IT FEEL LIKE?
These subtle muscles take concentration and practise to engage. You'll feel some burning but also a sense that you're twisting as the dominant movement (as opposed to leaning/squatting/bending).
CAUTION?
Our body is very injury prone when twisting and even more fragile when twisting and flexing. Ensure when you're twisting you keep tight through your obliques and conscious of the muscles working
MUST KNOW?
There is a rarely talked about secondary role of our twisting muscles and that is to occasionally avoid unwanted twisting. Say for example you're lifting a suitcase off an airport carousel, you're far safer staying strong and straight as you lift. However, this awkward lift can easily twist you into an awkward position. Your twisting muscles are responsible for twisting against the weight, so you stay straight.

04 extension

WHAT IS IT?
It's the exact opposite of spinal flexion. You start in a hunched posture with spine flexed then actively work against gravity to leave flexion and go into a neutral position or a safe hyper-extended position.
WHAT DOES IT TARGET?
It mainly targets the muscles that run along the spine in your lower back. However the hamstrings and gluteals also work to assist.
WHAT SHOULD IT FEEL LIKE?
If you're doing the neutral version (above) you want to feel this predominantly in hamstrings and glutes. With spinal flex and extend variations it's okay to feel in the muscles down the sides of your spine.
CAUTION?
For the vast majority of exercises feeling pain in your back is a problem. However, spinal extension is an exception. Just make sure you can decipher between joint pain (bad) and muscle pain (good).
MUST KNOW?
The lower back muscles are part of a team known as 'the posterior chain' along with the gluteals and hamstrings. A healthy back means these three working in unison when you're bending and lifting.

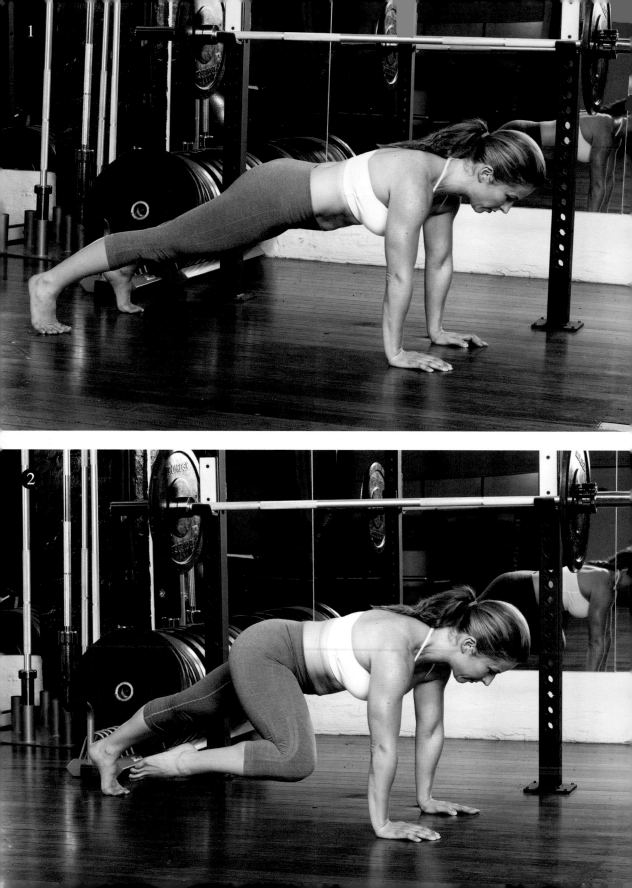

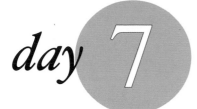
core climbers

MOVEMENT TYPE
BRACE TWIST

targets	BLACK	BLUE	RED
	100	70	40

why?
This takes the common bridge to the next level. While the bridge is a great exercise, the addition of movement creates more crossover benefits for real life.

how?
Start in a push up position with your feet shoulder-width apart, chest over hands, vision out in front of your hands and body in good posture. Now raise one foot and bring the knee in until your thigh reaches vertical. The key here is to move this leg in without rotating your hips and torso. By losing one of your supports your body wants to twist. By staying strong through your core you'll fight the tendency to twist and therefore maintain alignment.

your record

DATE				
level reached				

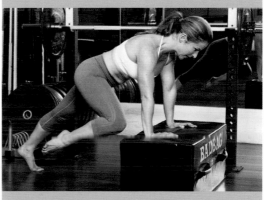

easier version

core climbers too hard? Rather than having your hands on the ground, place them on a raised bench.

Go through this move mindlessly and you'll get nothing out of it. Keep your focus and realise that even the slightest drop in your hips (even an inch) will reduce the effectiveness.

day 8

medicine ball twists

MOVEMENT TYPE
TWIST BRACE

targets

	BLACK	BLUE	RED
targets	200	175	100

why?
Our body is at its most fragile when we're twisting. If you consider most injuries, especially sports-related, there's often a twisting component to the stress. Hence why it's really important to strengthen ourselves against this weakness.

how?
Take a seat on the ground holding a medicine ball or other light weight (2-3kg is heaps). Sitting with good posture lower your torso back to 30 degrees. Maintain straight posture. To ensure your head is in the right position, imagine you're holding an apple between your chin and chest. Now you're in position for the twists. Starting with your ball 30cm from your stomach, twist your torso and rotate the ball to your left. Stop twisting when the ball reaches a few inches from the ground. Twist back to the start then onto the other side.

The trick with this exercise is to twist through your abs, not your hips. To do this focus on twisting at the level of your belly button, keep both bum cheeks evenly weighted on the ground and don't move your legs. If you feel your obliques (side abdominals) working you're on track.

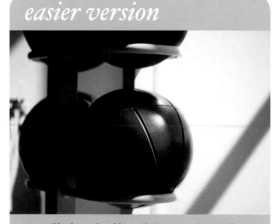

easier version

medicine ball twists too hard?
Do exactly the same move but pretend to hold weight. If this still is not appropriate for you, stand up and perform a twisting movement on the horizontal at waist height.

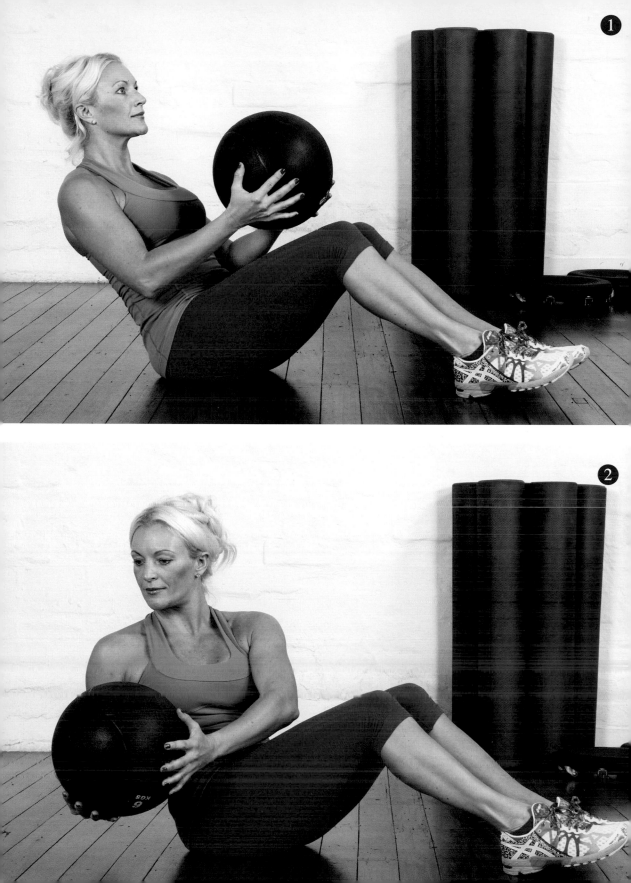

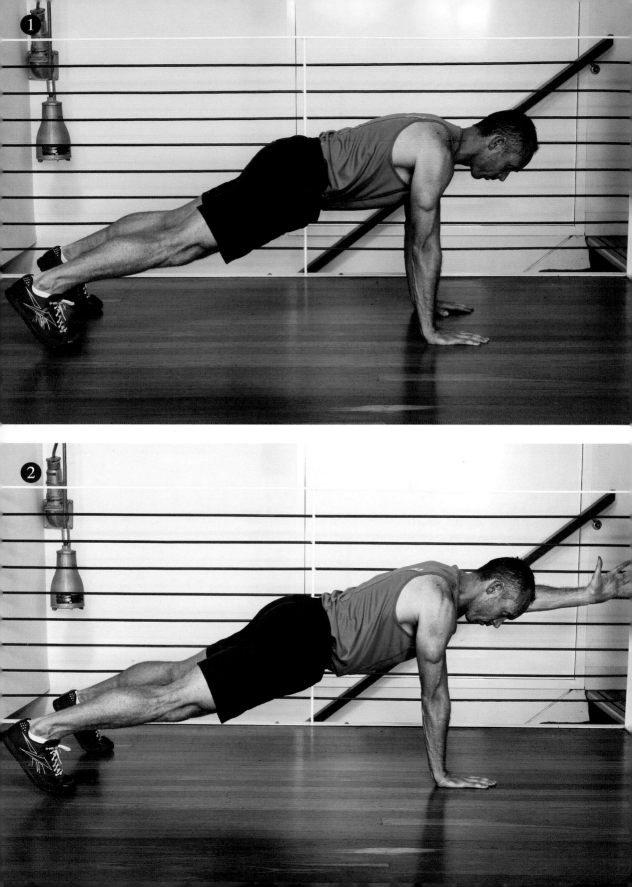

prone arm extensions

MOVEMENT TYPE
BRACE TWIST

targets	BLACK	BLUE	RED
	100	70	40

why?

Any prone exercise is a great way to strengthen your hip and core stability. Core strength has huge day-to-day movement benefits. This version ups the ante by requiring your body to perfectly stabilise while removing one of your supports.

how?

Assume a prone push-up position on your hands with arms vertical and body in one straight line. Have your foot just wider than shoulder width to give stability. It's important to strongly brace your stabilising core muscles so your hips are locked in place. Once your body is set rock solid, raise your right arm off the ground and reach it up and forward. By taking away one of your body's supporting pillars, you're forcing everything else to work harder to maintain a strong, stable position. Slowly lower the arm back to the ground and repeat with other arm.

As you do this movement imagine that I have rested a tray of champagne glasses on your back and your job is not to spill a drop.

your record

DATE				
level reached				

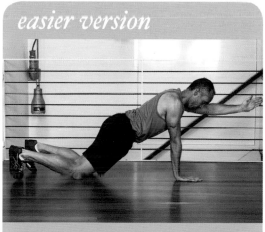

easier version

prone arm extensions too hard?
Try this on your knees or start with your hands on a raised surface like a bench.

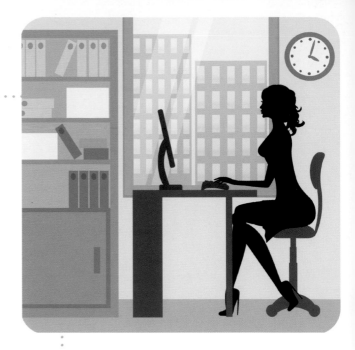

6 *triple flexion, triple threat*

problem:

While triple flexion sounds like a skill mastered by an agile circus performer, it's actually a term coined to describe our daily position when seated. You might be surprised to know that humans are not really designed to sit. Think back to our forefathers and foremothers and there wasn't a whole lot of sitting going on. Their constant movement was almost always upright.

The problem with sitting (other than the fact that it's not great for burning calories) is that your knees, hips and spine are generally all simultaneously flexed. This causes an unhealthy and unnatural shortening of some muscles and lengthening of others. Of particular concern is the flexion at the spine. Remember I earlier spoke about the soft s-shaped curve associated with good posture. Constant spinal forward flexion takes this preferred 'S' and turns it into an ugly 'C'. All the discs are squashed and their nutrients squeezed out. This can eventually lead to disc bulges and the like.

remedy:

Like most things with your body it craves balance. If you spend your day in unavoidable flexion you need to even the ledger by doing some extension. The easiest, do-anywhere version is the cobra (refer to page 22). Simply lie on your stomach, palms facing down under your shoulders and push up ensuring your hips bones stay grounded. Aim for 20 reps every day for improved disc health and to get your 'S' back.

7 *quality vs quantity*

I love challenges. I quickly get bored with workouts that don't test me or push me. So, the 30 Days of Abs challenge that fills these pages is going to be challenging for you regardless of your starting experience or strength. However, there is a but, isn't there always? Some of the daily challenges involve plenty of reps. Whenever possible try not to get into the mindset of just getting them done. With abs and core training in particular, quality always rules over quantity. If you rush through your reps or do too many at a time, your technique will suffer and you won't get the muscle adaptation I intend for you.

remember these rules:

If it's a flexing move it should burn; if it's an extension move you should feel it in your hammies, bum and a little in your back muscles; if it's a twisting move you should initiate and dominate the movement with your twisting muscles and finally, if it's bracing you need to fight to maintain perfect posture.

8 hey, sugar!

Refined sugar makes everything taste good - why is it bad for us?

Let's take a look at what's happening on the inside every time you have a sweet treat. Refined sugar is high in calories yet offers zero nutrition (commonly referred to as 'empty calories'). It also becomes destructive once consumed in excess, as our bodies can't break it down efficiently. Excess energy from refined sugar that is not metabolised in the body gets stored as fat around our important organs, like our liver and pancreas. This leads to a host of metabolic diseases, such as diabetes. So then, what does this look like on the outside? It looks like the little pot belly that you just can't shift. It's that last five kilos that won't go away. So, to make the most of your training, try limiting your sugar intake and feel the benefits.

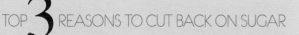

TOP 3 REASONS TO CUT BACK ON SUGAR

WEIGHT GAIN.
Sugar or glucose is energy for our cells. A sugar craving is the body asking for energy, however if we're eating too much of it, the excess energy is stored as fat and toxins.

IT'S HIGHLY ADDICTIVE.
The constant sugar roller coaster will wreak havoc on your blood sugar levels and hormones.

IT LEADS TO DISEASE.
As sugar consumption increases amongst us, so does obesity, heart disease and diabetes. Sugar addiction has also been linked to causing inflammation, depression, fatigue, skin irritations and poor digestion.

When reading food labels, 4g of sugar = 1 teaspoon, so aim for less than 6g of sugar per 100g serving of food.

HOW TO overcome sugar addiction

> Balance your blood sugar levels the right way, by eating a rainbow of fruit and vegetables. Include naturally sweet vegetables such as sweet potato, pumpkin, corn and peas.

> Drink plenty of water and make friends with sweetly scented herbal teas and pure coconut water.

> Use safer sweeteners in moderation, such as raw honey, pure maple syrup, rice malt syrup, unrefined green stevia and coconut products.

> Satiate your appetite by including protein and healthy fats with every meal and snack.

9 smooth operator

NUTRIENT DENSE SOUPS AND SMOOTHIES CAN REDUCE THE BURDEN ON YOUR DIGESTIVE SYSTEM. THEY ARE EASY TO PREPARE, LOW COST AND YOU CAN BE AS CREATIVE AND COLOURFUL AS YOU LIKE. MAKE SURE YOU ARE BUILDING YOUR SMOOTHIES AND SOUPS JUST LIKE YOU WOULD ANY OTHER MEAL, INCLUDING QUALITY CARBOHYDRATE, PROTEIN AND FAT. SEE THE RECIPE SECTION AT THE BACK OF THIS BOOK FOR INSPIRATION.

day 10

sit up with twist

MOVEMENT TYPE
SPINAL FLEXION TWIST

why?

I could talk fancy here or simply say I've combined two of the previous exercises into one. By doing that I'm adding complexity and giving you more bang for your buck.

how?

Sit holding a medicine ball (or equivalent weight) with your knees bent to 90 degrees, heels on the ground and torso tall. Lock your elbows into your ribs and hold the weight 20cm from your belly button. Now lower your torso back to the ground and stop once your shoulder blades touch the ground. Next, squeeze your abs and sit back up, flexing your tummy as you go. Once you reach a point approximately 10cm from upright, pause, then twist your torso first to the right and then left. Once you've twisted both ways, lower again and repeat. On each alternate rep twist the other way first to ensure balance. Try 3-5kgs for women and 4-8kgs for men.

If you use the weight to assist in propelling you up off the ground you're cheating. Be sure that you sit up purely due to the strength of your abs and not because you're using the ball to get you passed a sticking point.

your record

DATE				
level reached				

easier version

sit up with twist too hard?

Perform the same move with no weight

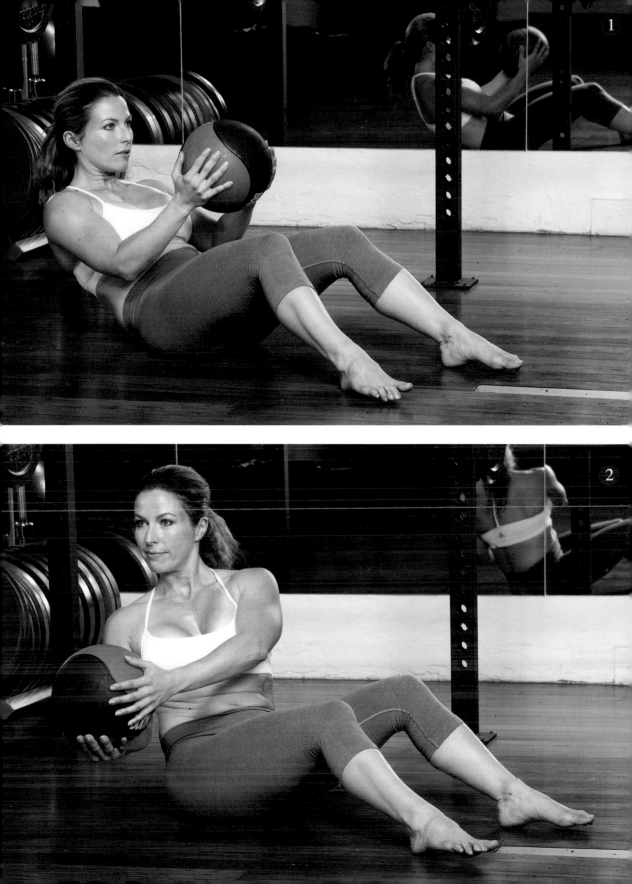

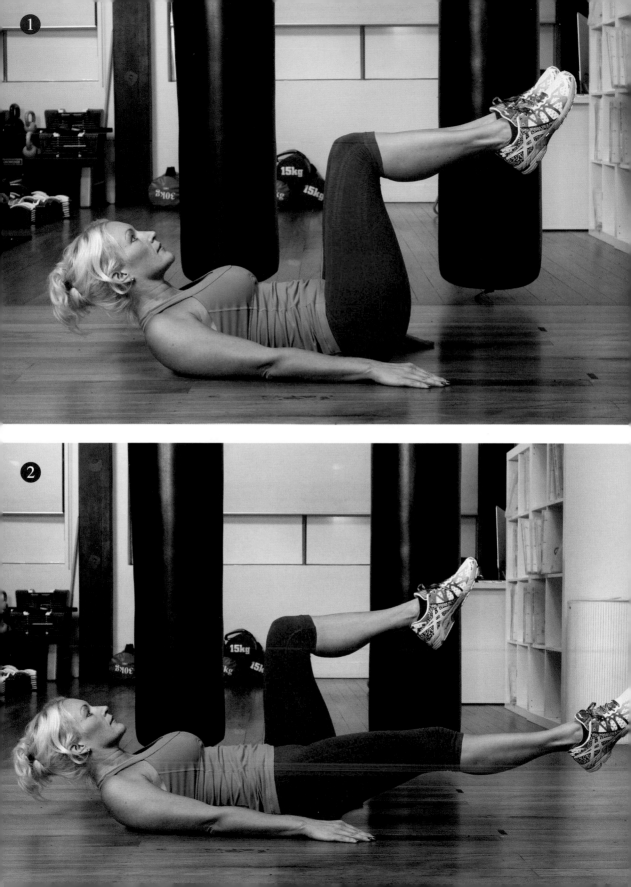

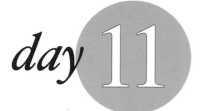

day 11

lying cycles

MOVEMENT TYPE
BRACE

why?
If you can get your abs to dominate this move it's a great little burner because your abs are having to control the demanding weight of your legs.

how?
Lie on your back on the ground. Raise both legs off the ground. Have your knees at 90 degrees, thighs vertical and your lower legs horizontal. Raise your head and shoulders off the ground so that your abs are ready to work. Now extend your right leg so that the heel finishes just off the ground and your leg is straight. Bring the leg back to where it started and repeat with your other leg.

You'll find far more success in recruiting your abs if you can get your thighs and hip flexors to switch off. Do this by pointing and wiggling your toes throughout.

your record

DATE				
level reached				

easier version

lying cycles too hard?
Perform the same move but reduce the range you extend your legs.

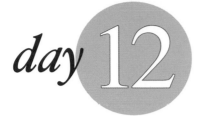
swiss ball back extensions

MOVEMENT TYPE
EXTENSION

targets	BLACK	BLUE	RED
	75	50	25

why?
It's important to balance out the obvious muscles we see in the mirror (and hence are motivated to train) and those usually hidden from view. You'll never hear someone say they want a ripped lower back but its strength is arguably more important than a ripped six-pack.

how?
Start by lying face down on top of a Swiss ball with the ball resting under your hips. Have your feet grounded and also lightly rest your fingers on the ground. Keeping the ball still, raise your torso up as high as you feel comfortable. You should feel your hamstrings engage, your glutes clench strongly and your lower back muscles working. Slowly lower back down over the ball, touch your fingers lightly to the ground and repeat.

your record

DATE				
level reached				

A smaller ball is best for this move. Also make sure it's properly inflated.

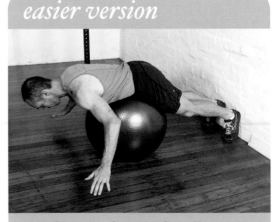

easier version

Back extension too hard?
Place ball under your stomach rather than hips so you aren't lifting as much of your weight. Gym access? Try a back extension machine to provide more stability.

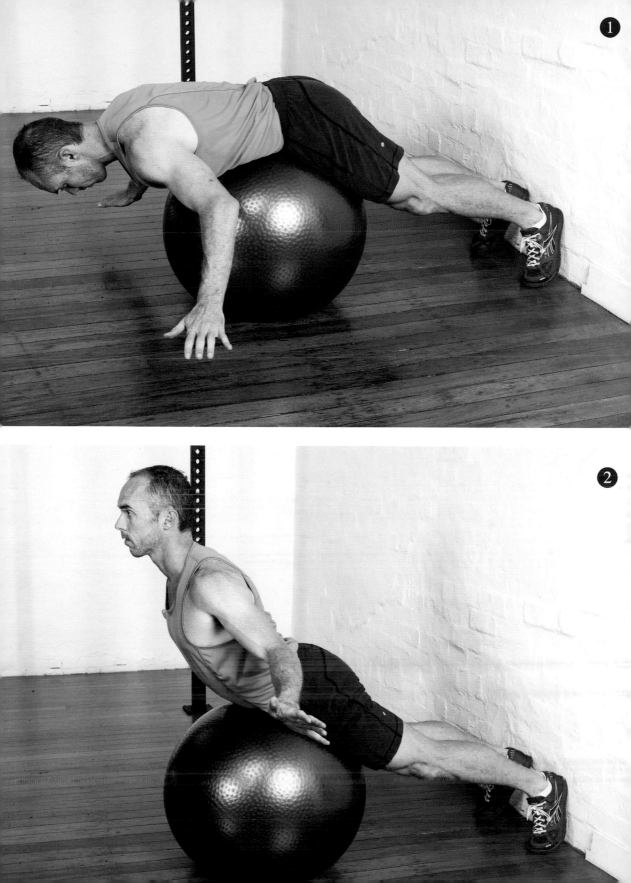

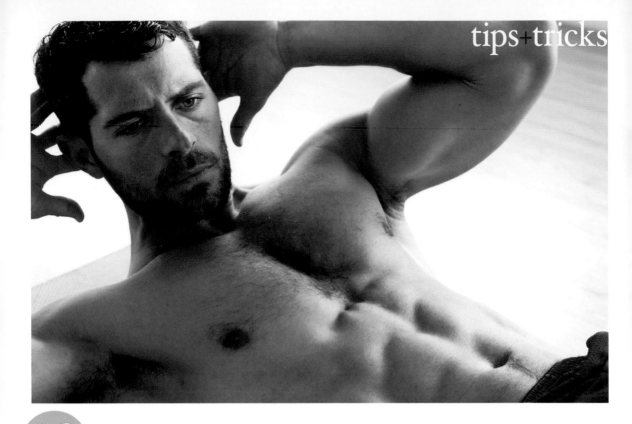

10 *the scale of determination*

How badly do you want to have the body of your dreams? How badly do you want noticeable definition in your abs? How badly do you want to have a body that is the envy of your friends?

The reality is most people will never achieve any of the above because they simply don't want it badly enough. But, you have an advantage. What you'll garner from this book is the ability to perform 30 moves with excellent technique.

However, if you want to see real change it's going to take more than that. It's going to take a reduction in your alcohol and sugar intake, regular and consistent training of high quality and a no-excuses attitude. If we break up the four main health and fitness goals, they're not all equal to achieve.

If you want to feel healthier - drink a little less alcohol, eat a little better, sleep a little more and be active more often (easy). If you want to be stronger and fitter, do the eating and sleeping thing better but ensure you're knocking out at least 2-3 high quality workouts out a week (easy-ish).

If you want to lose weight, you're going to need to ramp things up to the next level. Eating and drinking well most of the time. Training consistently and with purpose (pretty tough). But, if you want to have your abs peak through to

see daylight, arguably the hardest of all fitness goals, you're going to need to be very damn good. When you're offered a piece of birthday cake, you'll say no. When you're contemplating a mid-week drink. You'll say no. When you're struggling to get out of bed to get to the gym. You'll say hell yeah (very tough)

I'm not trying to deter you but I want you to be realistic. Not every goal is equal. Some will take bigger change, more willpower and more determination. But hey, you're up for the challenge aren't you?

12 *perk up*

Caffeine is the most consumed stimulant in the world and occurs naturally in plants such as the coffee bean, tea leaf and cocoa seed. Although limited intake of coffee, tea and dark chocolate can have some health benefits, consuming them too regularly will add unnecessary acidity to your body, affecting blood purification, liver function, sleep quality, overall hormone homeostasis and effective weight management. Too much caffeine also adds pressure on our adrenal system by producing excess cortisol, the 'stress' hormone - also referred to as the 'fat-grabbing' hormone. Instead of getting caught on the addictive rollercoaster of caffeine and artificial stimulants, rely on food and movement for real energy.

Good coffee & tea choices (1-2 cups a day and choose organic produce where possible):

> Long black with a sprinkle of ground cinnamon (almost no kilojoules and the cinnamon is a smooth, sweet addition without the blood sugar spike).

> Have full cream milk but make the coffee smaller (piccolo latte or small flat white).

> Be aware that black tea contains about half the caffeine of regular coffee. Most herbal teas contain no caffeine so try substituting black tea for peppermint, dandelion or ginger.

11 *wine time*

Whether you have a glass of wine every night with dinner, reserve drinking for the weekends or decide to completely binge every so often, consuming alcohol will set back any weight loss or healthy living regime. In a nutshell, for every gram of alcohol you consume 7 calories - about twice the amount per gram of carbohydrates and proteins. Not only are these calories likely to store as fat but there is no nutritional value in them - another form of 'empty calories'. What's more, with the slowing effect that it has on digestion, as well as the tendency it gives for increased appetite, alcohol makes for a seriously toxic weight-gain culprit. It's hard to maintain a lean physique if you let alcohol be your vice. If you must, limit alcohol consumption to special occasions only and follow these guidelines:

> Don't go crazy; just stick to 1-3 drinks per session.

> Up your water intake to counterbalance its dehydrating effects.

> Reduce calories and make your drink last longer by adding extra ice cubes to your glass.

> Avoid salty bar snacks as they will increase your alcohol cravings.

> Surround yourself with like-minded healthy people who enjoy activities other than drinking together.

> Avoid alcohol with heavy meals, and your digestion system will thank you.

13 A WORD ON SUGAR FROM DAMIEN

I'll happily let nutritionist Jasmine Sakr run the nutrition show in this book but I have one pearl of wisdom. I was born with a sweet tooth. My father has a sweet tooth and I'm pretty sure his dad did too. After dinner each night, I'd have a little sweet. I often caved in to a mid-morning sweet treat too. I was in my twenties, trained hard and smart so it didn't really matter so much. But by my thirties it started to matter. A little layer of insulation started to develop around my tummy and I could no longer be proud of my abs. I did one thing to turn this around. I gave up sweets for twelve months. The result was that with no noticeable change in my training I developed the best abs of my life. Sugar and alcohol can be the biggest barriers to having toned, head-turning abs.

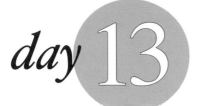
brazilians

MOVEMENT TYPE
BRACE TWIST

	BLACK	BLUE	RED
targets	100	70	40

why?

The core climber took the bridge to the next level and this does the same to the core climber. Adding rotation brings in even more muscles and makes it even more functional.

how?

Start in a push up position with your feet shoulder-width apart, chest over hands, vision out in front of your hands and body in good posture. Raise your right foot off the ground and draw your knee across and towards your opposite elbow.
The aim here is to stay long through your spine, so no hunching, but still try to twist your spine as much as you can. Your shoulders should remain over your hands and your head should stay in posture. Alternate feet on each rep.

The pace should be slow and each rep should take 3-4 seconds.

your record

DATE				
level reached				

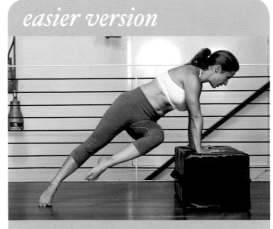

easier version

brazilians too hard? Start with your hands on a raised surface like a bench.

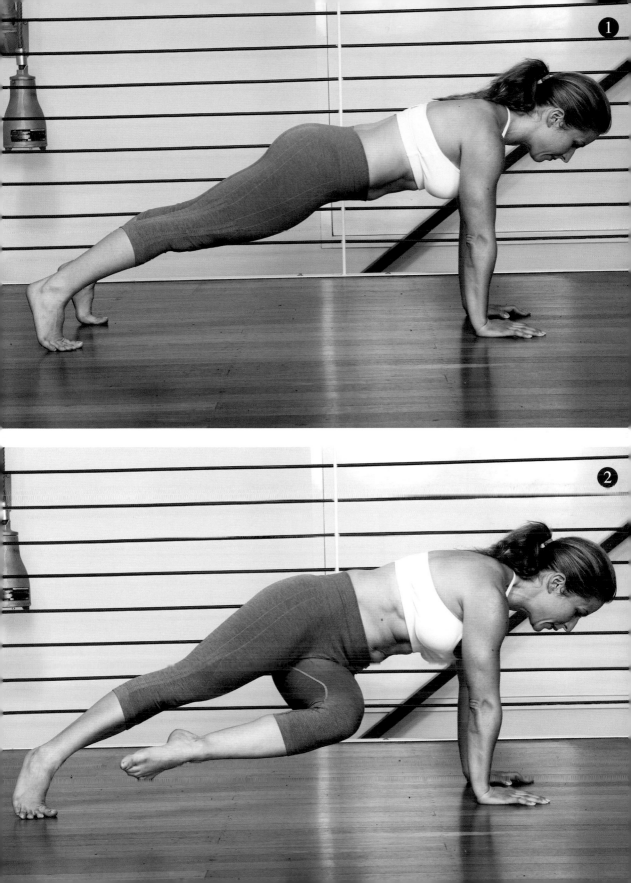

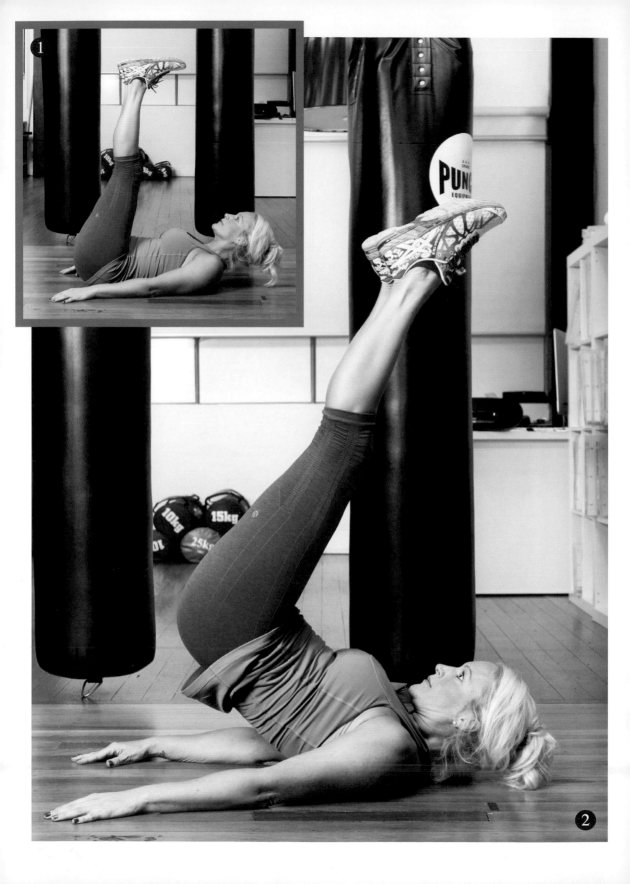

day 14

reverse crunch

MOVEMENT TYPE
SPINAL FLEXION

targets	BLACK	BLUE	RED
	100	70	40

why?

I generally don't favour partial range of motion moves like crunches but this version tends to work well at giving a great abs burn. A great burn means a hard-working muscle which equals awesome results.

how?

Lay on your back with your thighs vertical but knees slightly bent. Place your arms, palms down, on the floor beside you and have your head and shoulders off the ground. Now, squeezing through your abs raise your tailbone off the ground and move your feet up and above your head. Be careful not to use momentum. Control the down phase so that your hips don't crash back to the ground and go again.

As you lower your hips down during each rep the tendency is to allow your legs to go past vertical. If you do this your legs tend to swing up and into the next rep which greatly reduces the stress on the muscle.

your record

DATE				
level reached				

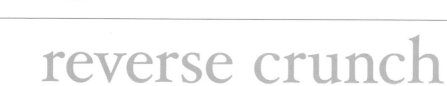

easier version

reverse crunches too hard? Bend your knees to ninety degrees throughout.

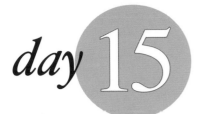
prone nose touches

MOVEMENT TYPE
BRACE

targets

	BLACK	BLUE	RED
targets	100	70	40

why?
This exercise has a dual purpose. Like a bridge it's a great core strengthener as your body fights gravity to stay straight. But the movement targets your lats and triceps, giving more results.

how?
Go down into a bridge position on your forearms and toes. Ensure your posture is straight and strong. Now bending at your elbows, allow your torso to move forward and touch your nose to the ground in front of your hands. Pull back up until you're back in the starting position.

your record

DATE				
level reached				

Squeeze your hands into fists so that your upper back is more easily locked into a strong and stable position.

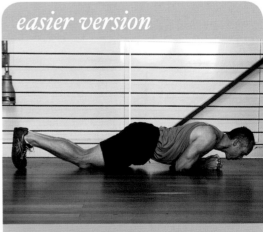

easier version

prone nose touches too hard?
Try this on your knees.

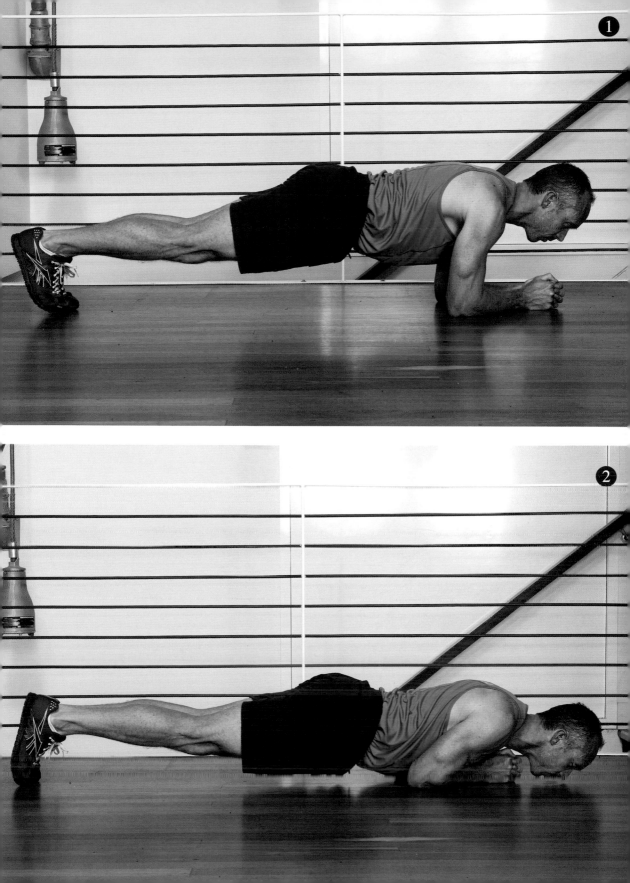

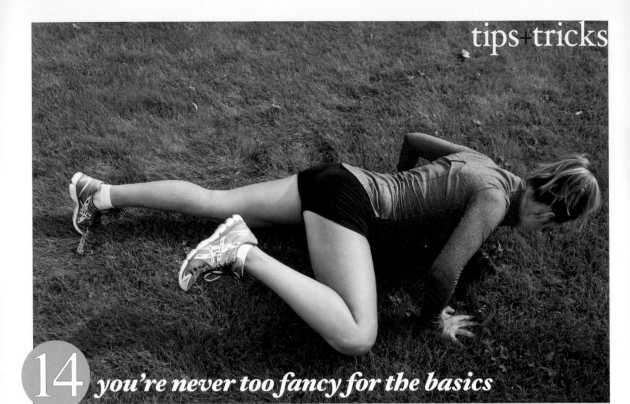

14 *you're never too fancy for the basics*

Yes, it can be cool to be fancy in the gym. Standing on a Swiss Ball with a barbell held overhead doing squats is ridiculously fancy, but it doesn't necessarily mean your body is working flawlessly. A great example is the injury-prone sports star. Yes, they can shoot hoops with staggering skill or break more tackles or run faster than a mere mortal. But, why are they always pulling a hamstring or getting back spasms? It's because they've moved too far away from being good at the basics.

Neglecting the basics can mean that all your big global muscles continue to improve but your super important deeper muscles may be faltering. What this means is that while your stack of cards is almost reaching the roof, the foundation is wobbly.

A good plan of attack is to schedule in some basic exercises every couple of weeks (or even add them to every warm-up) so that your foundations of movement are strong. The way I've structured the 30 day of Abs Challenge is that they progressively get harder as you move through. So, be conscious that once you finish this challenge you continue to practise and perfect the moves from the first ten days, just as much as you continue to challenge yourself with the fun fancy moves.

15 GOING THROUGH THE MOTIONS

I have another little exercise for you. Bend your arm at your elbow to 90 degrees. Now look at your biceps. The muscle should be relatively floppy as even though it has worked to get the arm to bend it hasn't had to work anywhere near it's maximum. Okay, straighten your arm. Now bend your arm again but this time imagine you are in a bodybuilding competition. In other words make the muscle flex as much as you can. Functionally, you've done the same thing both times (you've bent your elbow). The point of this little exercise is to highlight light and maximal muscle engagement. Sometimes you can fall into the trap of going through the motions. Say for example you are doing a sit up. Doing them without thinking means you go through the motion but have you properly and effectively engaged the muscle? Do a rep and consciously and strongly squeeze your abs and you'll have no doubt they're working. Also, because they are working so strongly you'll negate the chance of other more dominant muscles, like hip flexors in the sit up, taking over and ruining your results.

DID YOU KNOW? SUPER SEEDS LIKE CHIA AND GROUND LINSEEDS (FLAXSEED) ARE EXCELLENT FIBRE BOOSTERS, AS THEY SWELL AND ACT LIKE A "BINDING JELLY" FOR THE FOOD IN YOUR DIGESTIVE SYSTEM.

16 shredding and sculpting

Shredding and sculpting are terms that get plenty of airplay online. By taking on this 30 day challenge you will definitely build strength and definition around your mid-section. Especially if you're technique quality is high and you choose the appropriate levels. However, this program is not likely to help you drop body fat. The two best ways to do that are strength circuits and high intensity interval training.

A strength circuits involves you picking 2-5 'unlike' strength exercises and circuiting your way through them for approximately 10-15 reps each for 3-5 rounds. This is the king of training because it gets your heart rate up and causes the muscles to become hungrier. The two best fat devourers combined. Aim for three workouts per week and mix the exercises and format up often.

High Intensity Interval Training (H.I.I.T) is the most time efficient version of cardio. It involves consecutive intervals of hard work followed by rest. The harder the work (within reason), the better. The work to rest ratio is generally 2:1 but can be tweaked for the sake of variety. You can choose any form of cardio but generally it's wise to mix this up too. Don't just choose the things you're good at. You'll often burn more fat doing things you're bad at as you'll be less efficient. Check out my first book 'The Little Book of Big Workouts' for 31 great workout ideas to get you started, at damienkelly.com.au These workouts drop body fat and increase muscle so you can see muscle tone and definition.

17 soda stream

Think you're doing a good thing by swapping sugary soft drinks for diet versions? Reconsider, because diet sodas contain potentially harmful artificial sweeteners and chemicals and offer zero nutrition. Diet drinks are unlikely to be the direct cause of weight gain, however drinking them can often lead to overeating. Nutritionists speculate that diet drinks disrupt our body's ability to learn associations between sweet tastes and actual calories in food. So, although you think you may be satisfying a sweet craving by gulping a diet soda, you are only confusing your body into a fake sensation. This means that you will crave 'real' energy later, leading to uncontrolled meal portions and surplus snacking.

3 steps to giving up diet soda

step one: Evaluate your cravings.
Do you really desire that cola or is your body dehydrated? Reach for a glass of water first, then think about whether you truly want the soft drink.

step two: Still craving soda? Often it is the cold, numbing sensation that is the biggest temptation so experiment with having your soda warm instead. When your tongue is not numb, you will be able to decipher the real taste of what you're drinking.

step three: Introduce more water, herbal tea, coconut water and freshly prepared vegetable juices to your diet. Your soda cravings are bound to drop off in no time!

18 FEEL THE BURN

Yes, it's a bit 80's cringe to say 'feel the burn' but occasionally it's very important. If you're doing a plank, there is a fair chance you won't feel a burn. If you're doing a medicine ball twist, the chances are you won't smell smoke. But, if you are doing an exercise that involves your six-pack muscles, I want your shirt to catch fire, I want you to dial for a fire engine and call for water. Why? The abs will burn if they're working. They will complain so much that you're never in any doubt that they are working hard. So as per tip 15, squeeze them hard to ensure they're working and do as many as you can to get the full effect.

30KG

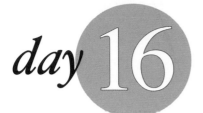

day 16

standing side flexion

MOVEMENT TYPE
SIDE FLEXION

	BLACK	BLUE	RED
targets	60e	40e	20e

why?

If you do this exercise properly, you'll feel it for about 48 hours post-workout. I've always found this move, due to the simultaneous stretching and strengthening, causes a fair amount of post workout soreness. In general, when isolated to the muscles, this is a good thing.

how?

Stand holding a weight (5-10kg for women and 10-20kg for men) in your left hand. Now, slide the weight down the outside of your leg. Do this by laterally flexing your spine. Lock your right hip in position and as you lower feel a stretch between your right hip and lower ribs. Once you've reached maximal stretch pause and rise slowly. On the up phase focus on squeezing and crunching your right side muscles.

your record

DATE				
level reached				

Lateral spinal flexion requires some caution. If you have a history of back injury or experience spinal discomfort during this move cease doing it and seek advice.

easier version

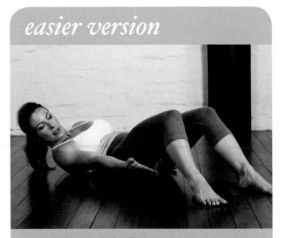

standing side flexion too hard?
Lie on your back with your feet on the ground. Bend your knees to ninety degrees with arms by your sides. Reach around with your right hand and try to touch your right heel then do the same on your left. You'll be doing the same style of side flexion but with your back supported.

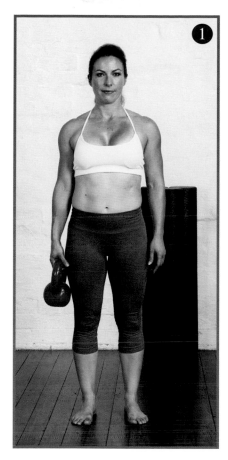

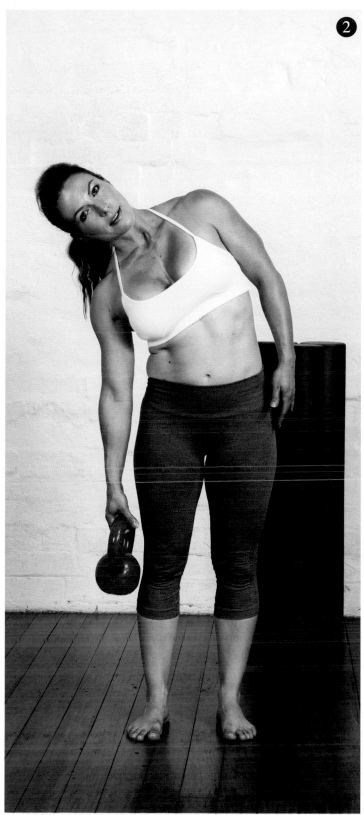

> IF YOU DO THIS EXERCISE PROPERLY, YOU'LL FEEL IT FOR ABOUT 48 HOURS POST-WORKOUT

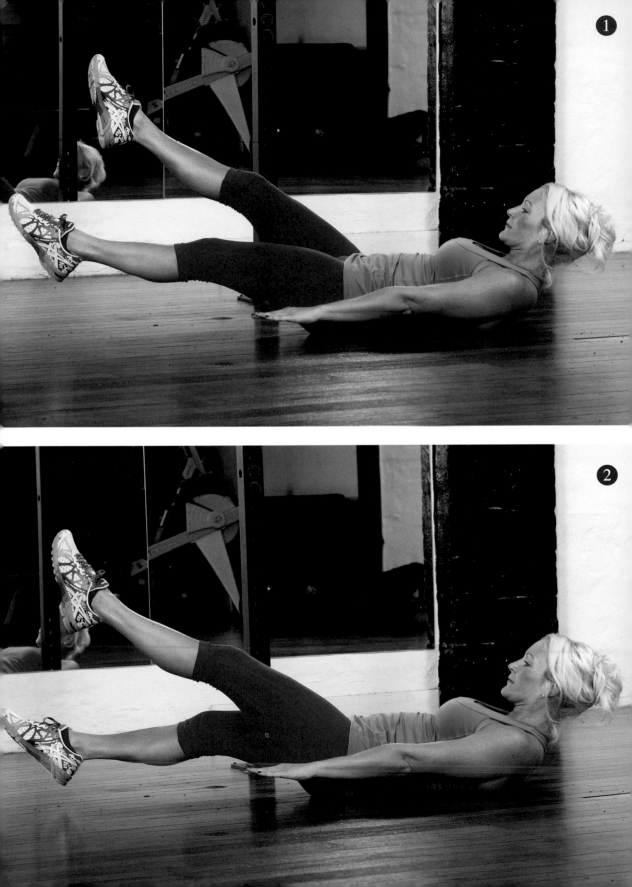

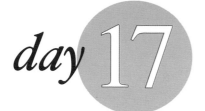

day 17

lying leg flutters

MOVEMENT TYPE
BRACE

targets	BLACK	BLUE	RED
	200	150	100

why?

You're creating a strong challenge when your abs must work against the weight of your legs. Having your legs close to the ground and straight makes this a very effective move.

how?

Lie on your back with your arms (palms down) beside your body and your legs out straight. Lift your head and shoulders off the ground to engage your abs. Point your toes then lift both legs a little off the ground. Now simultaneously raise your right leg and lower your left leg until they're about 20 cm apart. Next lower your right leg and raise your left leg until once again they're about 20 cm apart. Continue to flutter them in this fashion whilst trying to maintain a soft curve in your back (i.e. not flattening or over-arching).

I've mentioned in a few exercises to point your toes. This is a nice trick to ensure that your abs and not your legs are the prime movers in the exercise.

your record

DATE				
level reached				

easier version

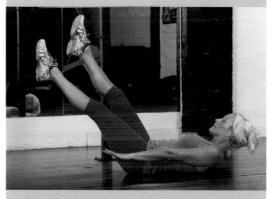

leg flutters too hard? Rather than have your legs fluttering near the horizontal line have them fluttering near the vertical line.

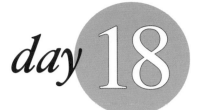

V sit ups

MOVEMENT TYPE
SPINAL FLEXION BRACE

targets	BLACK	BLUE	RED
	100	70	40

why?

This is numero uno when it comes to no-equipment six-pack exercises. It's tough, effective and it burns. The combination of controlling both upper and lower body simultaneously makes this move special.

how?

Sit on your backside, knees at 90 degrees and torso long and straight. Raise your feet off the ground and bring your thighs towards your chest. This move has you simultaneously extending your legs out towards the ground and lowering your torso to the ground. Stop just before either touches the ground. Flexing through your abs, sit up again and raise your legs, so that you finish once again with thighs into your chest.

your record

DATE				
level reached				

If you simply go through the motions you'll be missing a great opportunity, so control the pace of lowering. Make sure you also flex, crunch and squeeze your abs on the way up.

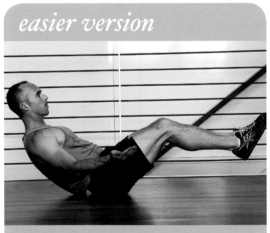

easier version

V sit ups too hard? You can simply reduce the range of motion or place your fingertips under your thighs to assist.

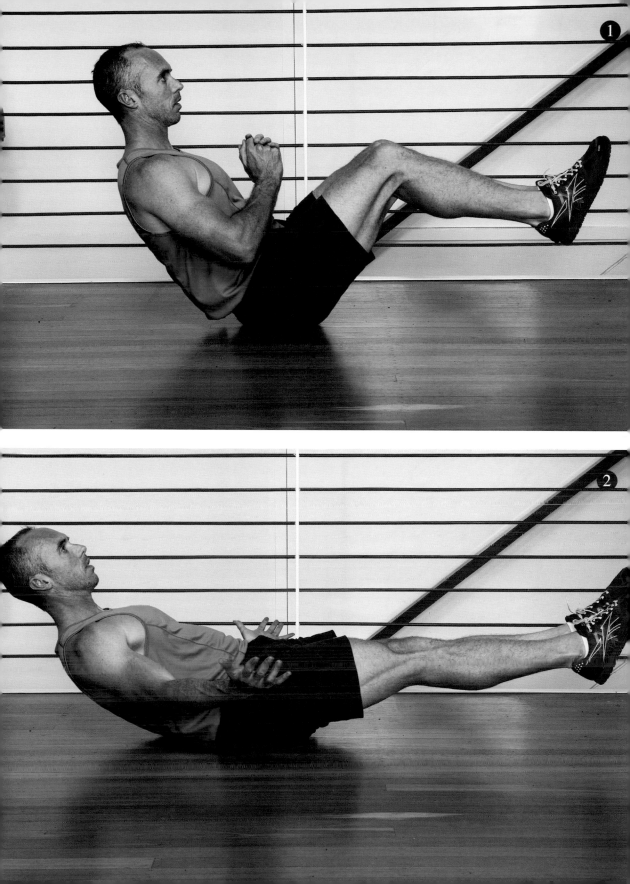

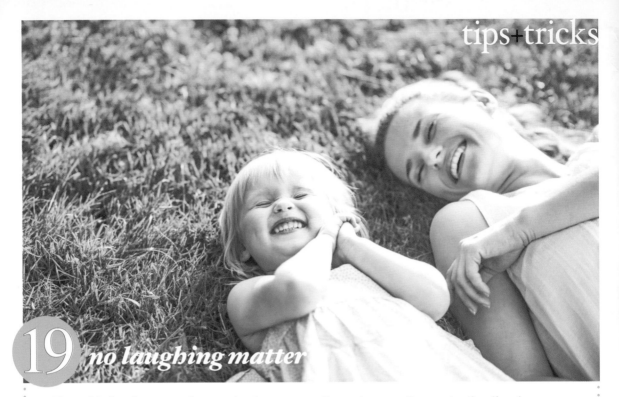

19 *no laughing matter*

Your pelvic floor is an area of your body you'll never give a second thought to until it becomes weak or ineffectual. Post-childbirth is the key time when the pelvic floor muscles can become problematic. The pelvic floor makes up the bottom section of your core. A weakness in the pelvic floor can literally cause a collapse in the bottom of this core 'box' (see Tip 22). The easiest way to engage your pelvic floor is to think of drawing up your nether region. For guys think 'nuts to guts'. to the bathroom. You'll notice it feels like a pulling up through your groin. And this is what a healthy pelvic floor does: pull up to support the bottom structure of the box.

If you are bearing down as you train your core, you're making the job of the pelvic floor infinitely harder. Instead start with some basic core exercises that allow you to practise proper pelvic floor contraction. If you're a new mum and having issues - rest easy, you're not the only one. My first big bit of advice is don't go too hard too soon. If you're doing exercises that your pelvic floor can't handle, it will only become weaker. Every time you're at a set of red lights or on the phone consciously perform pelvic floor contractions. Even if you're not currently experiencing weakness these exercises will still hold you in good stead.

20 THE QUALITY BREAKFAST

We've all been told not to skip breakfast. But what's the point of adhering if we are only consuming sugary cereals and boring toast with very little nutritional benefit? It's time we re-phrase that notion to: 'a QUALITY breakfast is the most important meal of the day'. Rethink what breakfast means to you. Who says you can't have your vegetables in the morning? Whatever you choose, start your day with a perfect balance of good carbohydrates, proteins and fats. Remember, carbs are our body's preferred energy source and come from anything that grows in the ground, especially vegetables and fruits. Protein keeps us full and is important for muscle repair and growth. Good fats are essential for brain function and healthy weight maintenance. If you begin your day well, chances are you will reduce cravings and make better food choices for your following snacks and meals. Check out the breakfast ideas in the recipe section of this book.

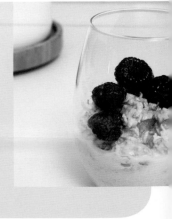

21 *fibre 101*

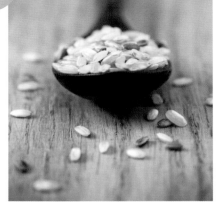

Eating enough fibre will keep your 'engine' clean and your body well fuelled. If we have great digestion, then we're more likely to maintain healthy weight, stay fuller for longer, remove toxins from our system and feel less bloated and more energetic.

Here are some simple ways to include adequate amounts of fibre in your diet - aim for at least 30 grams a day.

vege out!
Make vegetables the staple part of your diet. Include varied types of veggies with as many meals as possible - there should be more on your plate than anything else.

bean there
Add beans and legumes to your meals.

swap it
Swap high energy, calorie dense snacks & sweets for fruits & vegetables.

skip juice
Eat whole fruits instead of fruit juice, which strips all fibre and leaves pure fructose only. Berries, apples and pears are great high fibre choices.

good start
Start your day with good quality oats, porridge or muesli topped with nuts, seeds and fresh fruit.

the white stuff
Ditch refined white stuff and go for whole grains all the way, for example, brown rice, wholemeal, rye and quinoa.

22 *breath yourself a six-pack*

You now know the core is made up of your TVA muscle and obliques but the structure of your core is actually more like a box that sits in your lower torso. The sides of the box are made up of the TVA, obliques and some back muscles. The top of your box is your diaphragm and the bottom of your box is your pelvic floor. It's the ability to brace this entire system that allows for ultimate core strength. You may brace your TVA and obliques but if you're breathing the wrong way, the system may still be weakened by the diaphragm. The breathing required for a strong diaphragm takes practise but it's best described as breathing through pursed lips. This allows necessary breath in and out without a loss in intra-abdominal pressure. On the other hand, holding your breath can cause too much pressure. Of particular importance is when you're doing spinal flexion. These moves reduce the space of the abdominal area so you need to breathe out as you're flexing. Once again through pursed lips to maintain the adequate pressure.

23 THE RIGHT FATS

The word is out - (the right) fats don't make you fat. In fact, sensible fats are essential and contribute to satiety, optimal organ function and weight management. Low fat and diet products are often loaded with sugar for taste and can lead to overeating. Choose whole, unprocessed, full-fat versions in lesser quantities. If you're trying to slim down, limit added fats to 10% of meals and snacks.

GOOD FATS	SAY NO TO...
Avocado	Vegetable oils (including soy, corn and canola)
Organic grass-fed butter and ghee	
Coconut oil and unprocessed coconut products.	Trans fats & hydrogenated oils
Extra virgin olive oil and whole olives	Margarine
Oily fish, (salmon, sardines)	
Nuts, particularly walnuts plus nut oils and butters, like peanut and macadamia	
Seeds, like flaxseed plus seed oils (like sesame and grapeseed)	

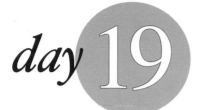

day 19

mountain jumpers

MOVEMENT TYPE
BRACE

targets	BLACK	BLUE	RED
	100	70	40

why?

Often life happens quickly without prior notice. That's when our training shows its true function - allowing us to switch on our muscles in a fraction of a second. Pure strength is lovely but being able to switch on muscles when needed is even sweeter.

how?

Assume a push-up position in perfect posture. Keeping your hands where they are, jump both feet in towards your hands. On landing your knees will be tucked in towards your chest. Hold for a second then jump your legs back out again. This is the key part of the exercise. When jumping out your goal is to lock your body into perfect posture on the first attempt. You shouldn't let your hips sag. Once you've held this posture for a couple of seconds, start your next rep.

This is another move where it's nice to have another set of eyes on you. You may not feel a slight drop of the hips on landing but a partner will. Utilise a mirror if you don't have a training partner.

your record

DATE				
level reached				

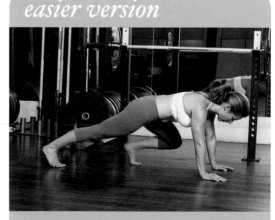

easier version

moutain jumpers too hard?
Step your feet out rather than jump out. Be conscious of finishing in a perfectly straight and strong prone position.

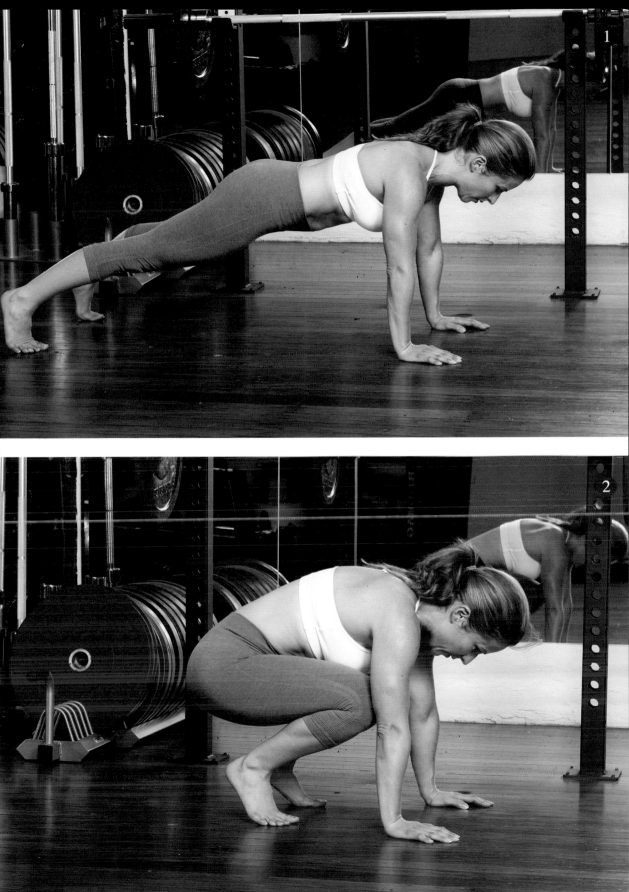

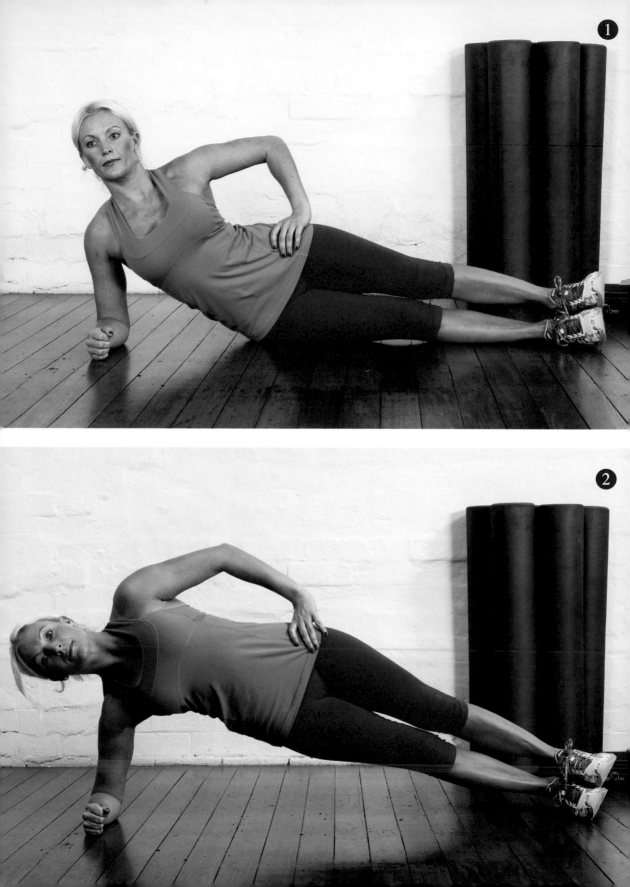

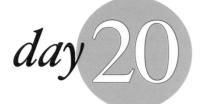

day 20

side bridge

MOVEMENT TYPE
BRACE TWIST

why?
The muscles colloquially called love handles are not only super functional for daily movement but also rather sexy when on show. This move is a great shaper and toner.

how?
Lie on your side with your body straight, leaning on your elbow, with your forearm pointing forward. Have your knees straight and feet stacked on top of each other. Brace your core, front and sides. To do this imagine a large belt has been tied around your waist and is being pulled to reduce the circumference of your abs. Raise your hip off the ground to form a straight line, from shoulder to knee. Ensure your head is in posture.

targets
(each side)

	BLACK	BLUE	RED
	3 min	2 min	1 min

your record

DATE				
level reached				

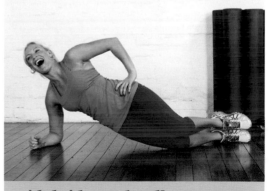

easier version

side bridge too hard? You've got three options: rest on your knees rather than feet; raise your forearm position onto a bench or place your top hand on the ground throughout.

Throughout the move continue to push your hips up and forward to ensure the the right muscles are firing correctly.

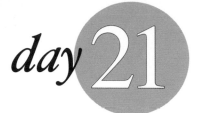

swiss ball supermans

MOVEMENT TYPE
BRACE TWIST

targets	BLACK	BLUE	RED
	100	80	60

why?
Once again strength is not the only key core attribute. Being able to switch your core muscles on as soon as you need them is equally important. This will forever protect your back and have you moving faster and stronger.

how?
Lie with your stomach on the ball with fingertips on the ground in front and your toes on the ground out back. Brace your core muscles to stop the ball pushing into your stomach and to steady your body against the instability. Have your head in neutral and spine long. Simultaneously raise your right hand and left foot off the ground and raise up until the arm and leg are horizontal. Hold for a couple of seconds then lower with foot and fingertips grounding again simultaneously. Next raise opposite arm and leg.

The tendency in this move is to raise the hand slightly before the foot. This makes the exercise far easier and should be avoided. Be careful to raise the hand and opposite leg at exactly the same time to maximise results.

your record

DATE				
level reached				

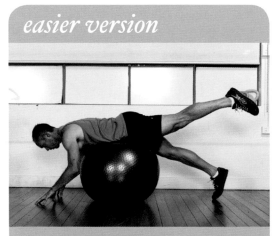

easier version

supermans too hard? Cheat this move and do exactly what I just said not to. Raise your hand first and then your opposite foot, pause, lower then repeat on the other side.

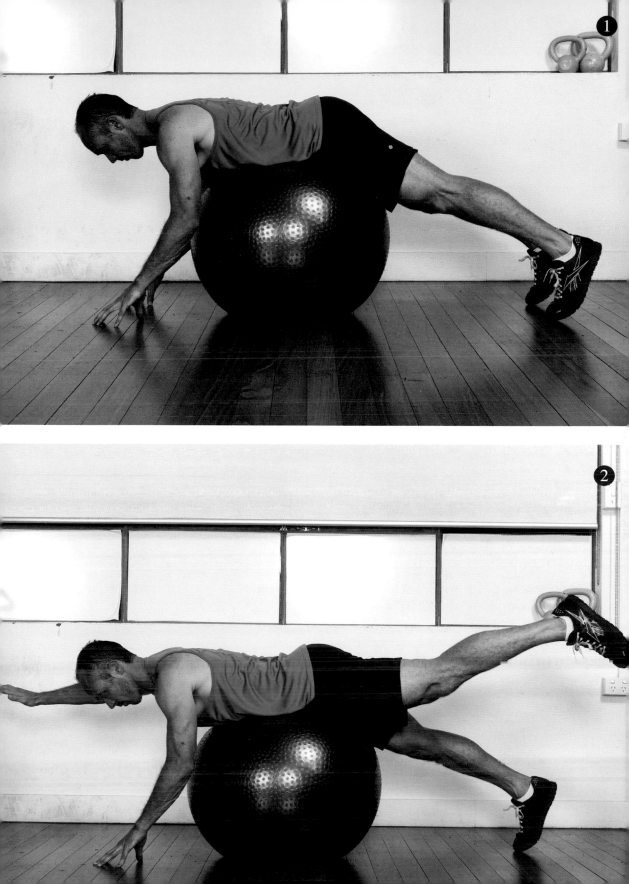

24 *core business*

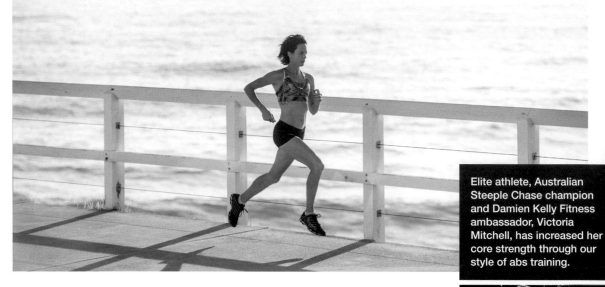

Elite athlete, Australian Steeple Chase champion and Damien Kelly Fitness ambassador, Victoria Mitchell, has increased her core strength through our style of abs training.

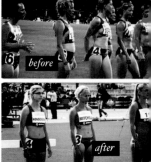

before

after

A very smart physio friend of mine, Anna-Louise Bouvier, developed a chart on the hierarchy of core training. The premise was that the most basic moves were at the start and it moved step by step through progressively harder exercises. The point she makes is that not all core exercises are created equal and that you must master the basic moves before you progress to the more advanced moves. The theory being that if you do a move that you're not really ready for you're not going to be engaging your core properly and are therefore at best reducing the benefit of the exercise and at worst increasing the risk of injury. That's why I want you to really focus on mastering the techniques in the early part of my program.

If you don't feel like you've mastered an exercise, pause the program, repeat the exercise and hopefully you'll master it second time around. Alternatively move through making notes on which exercises need particular work in the future.

25 GOOD SPORT

At the top of Bouvier's core hierarchy was dynamic sporty-type movements. The reason is that as soon as you add speed and complexity to a movement it is harder for a muscle to time the appropriate contraction. It's often why injuries occur and plays a part in why some people are more athletic than others. When it comes to running, core training is oh so important. If you watch an elite runner they have amazing control through their core, making them so strong and stable. This allows for all their efforts to go directly into helping them move forward. A weak core will mean that the movement of the upper body will affect the lower body as it's not able to dampen the rotation. The result is that rather than solely being concerned about propelling you forward they are also needing to deal with unwanted rotation and useless movement. A great trick when you're running is to think tall. This has a couple of benefits. Firstly, being tall makes you feel better and more positive when you run. Secondly, being tall allows for your core to more easily engage. Lastly being tall helps your stride by allowing more length.

main image: marceau photography

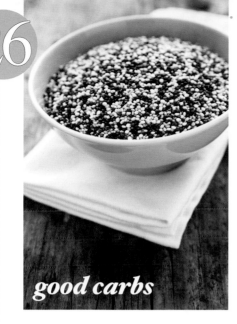

good carbs

Thanks to diet crazes of recent times, we've come to think of all carbohydrates as weight gain culprits. However, we need to be clear about the differentiation between bad and good forms of grain carbohydrates - that is, refined versus whole grains. There's no question that over-consumption of processed white breads, pastas and rice should be avoided due to their low nutrient density and ability to quickly turn into glycogen and body fat. On the reverse, whole and unrefined carbohydrates burn slowly in our systems and provide us with the lasting energy needed to be able to exercise, breathe, maintain healthy heart function and satiate our appetites. The best carbohydrate options include whole grains (e.g. oats, barley, brown rice), seeds (like quinoa), beans and most vegetables and fruits. Remember, traditional diets from around the world have always been based around great grains, so you can still have them but choose wisely.

EXPERIMENT WITH USING GRAIN ALTERNATIVES, LIKE SWAPPING SANDWICH WRAPS AND TACO SHELLS FOR CRISPY, FRESH LETTUCE LEAVES.

safe snacking

Be prepared and you'll never need the vending machine again! Keep cravings at bay with the right snacks that will keep you satiated between meals and keep your blood sugar levels balanced throughout the day. Remember, only eat snacks if you are hungry, not from boredom or habit. Some simple suggestions are:

> *A boiled egg and a small banana*

> *A handful roasted unsalted nuts (keep in your gym bag or handbag at all times) and a coconut water*

> *1 cup non-artificial, natural protein smoothie - available online or health food shops*

> *Protein bliss balls - see recipe page 89*

> *A handful of berries with unsweetened Greek yoghurt and a light sprinkling of seeds*

> *Veggie sticks with hummus or sugar-free nut butter*

> *DIY trail mix - use your favourite nuts and seeds to create your personalised snack. Add coconut chips and sulphur-free dried fruits for some sweet satisfaction. Also see recipe section of this book for inspiration.*

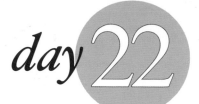

lying leg lowers

MOVEMENT TYPE
BRACE

	BLACK	BLUE	RED
targets	60	40	20

why?
Another of our core moves where your legs act as the weight. By keeping your legs straight you are forcing the abs to control a weight that is a long way away from the fulcrum. This makes the move exceptionally tough and exceptionally effective.

how?
Lie on your back with your hands, palms down, by your sides. Raise your legs up so that they are vertical. Raise your head and shoulders off the ground to help set a strong tummy. Lower your legs slowly towards the ground. The point at which you stop is determined by your strength. If you feel your back excessively arch or flatten, you have lowered too far. Raise your legs back to vertical.

If you stay tense and locked through feet and ankles, your hip flexors are going to dominate this move. By pointing and wiggling your toes you'll be forcing those lazy abs to play a bigger role.

your record

DATE				
level reached				

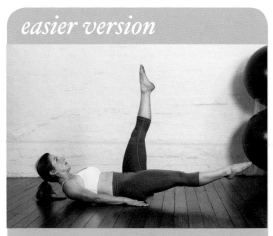

easier version

leg lowers too hard? Follow the same protocol but instead only lower one leg at a time.

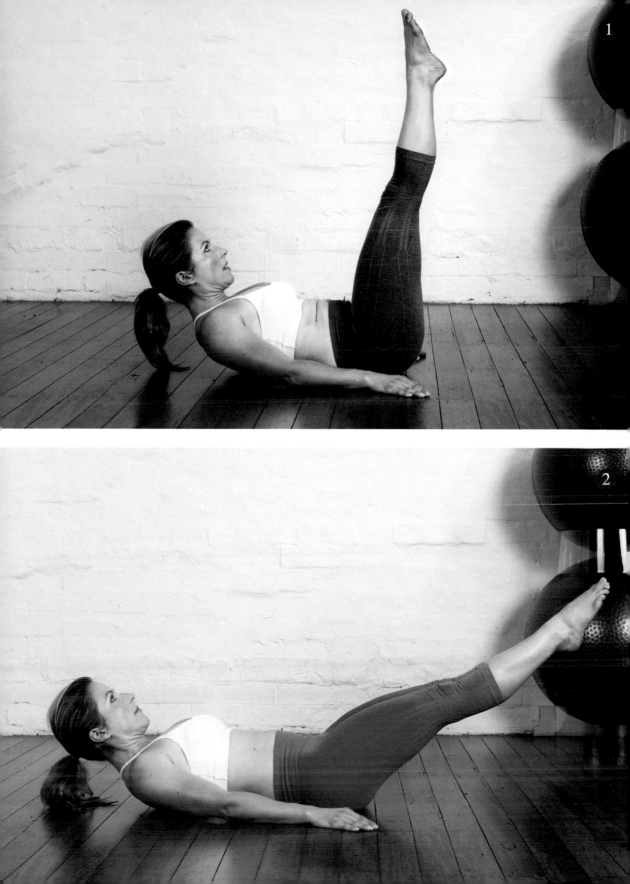

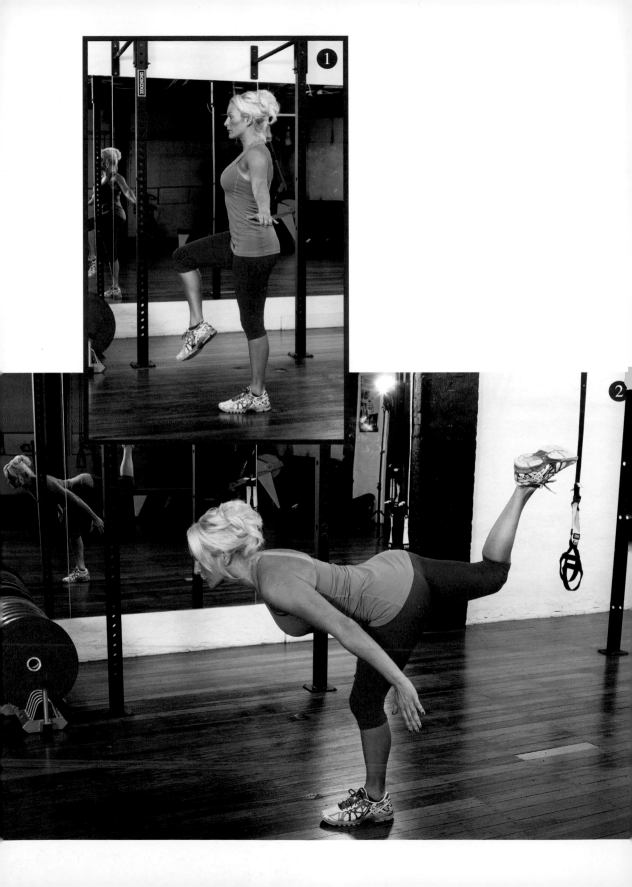

cranes

MOVEMENT TYPE
EXTENSION

why?

The deadlift is one of the top few most important moves you can do. It works all the important muscles of your posterior - think hamstrings, glutes and lower back. The crane is the one leg version to ensure both sides are strengthening equally. While not a 'classic' abs exercise, it earns its place here to balance the otherwise predominance of anterior focussed movements.

how?

Balance on one leg and place both hands out to your sides. Keeping the knee of your grounded leg almost straight, bend forward at your hips and lower your torso slowly to horizontal. As you do this your airborne leg will extend up and back until it also becomes horizontal. Aim to keep your back long and straight throughout by looking forward and keeping your chest open. You should feel this in the hamstring of the grounded leg.

Doing this in front of a mirror will ensure your symmetry is where it needs to be. Watch that your shoulders and hips stay level. Also keep lowering until you see your airborne foot raise above and beyond your horizontal torso.

	BLACK	BLUE	RED
targets (each side)	50	40	30

your record

DATE				
level reached				

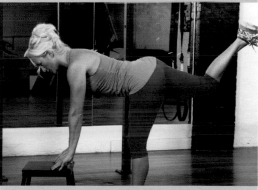

easier version

cranes too hard? Follow the same 'how' protocol but use a bench to stabilise your balance at the bottom of the move.

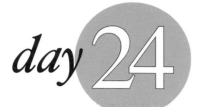

day 24

wipers

MOVEMENT TYPE
TWIST

why?
As I've said, when you utilise the weight of your legs (as opposed to an exercise like a sit up that utilises the weight of your torso) you are really upping the challenge. This is the first of your exercises using the legs to challenge the twist.

how?
Lie on your back with arms, palms down, spread out perpendicular from your torso. Raise your legs up into the air so that your feet are pointing to the sky. Your knees should have a slight bend in them. Brace your abs firmly and ensure that your arms are prepared to provide support. Slowly lower your legs to the side, whilst trying to keep your opposite shoulder grounded. Lower as far as you can whilst maintaining complete control. You should feel this strongly in your obliques on the side you are twisting away from. Lift your legs back up to the starting position and repeat on other side.

This exercise really needs your concentration to ensure that your twisting muscles are getting isolated. On the way down you should specifically feel the obliques stretching yet controlling the movement. At the bottom of the lowering, pause, then consciously engage your obliques to twist your legs back to vertical.

	BLACK	BLUE	RED
targets	100	74	50

your record

DATE				
level reached				

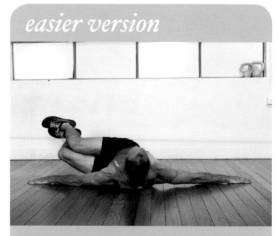

easier version

wipers too hard? Perform a similar twisting and lowering of your legs as the main exercise but instead maintain an exact 90 degree bend in your knees throughout.

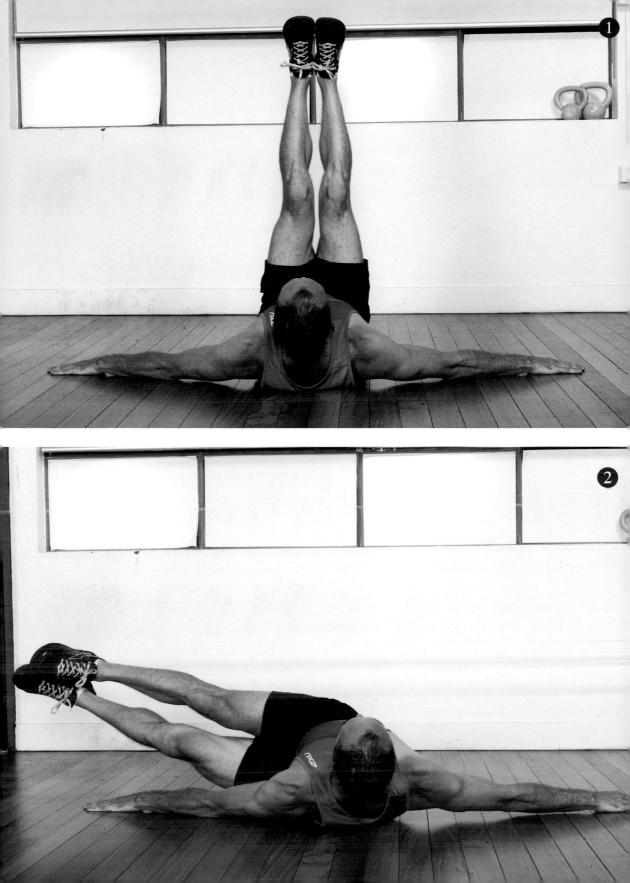

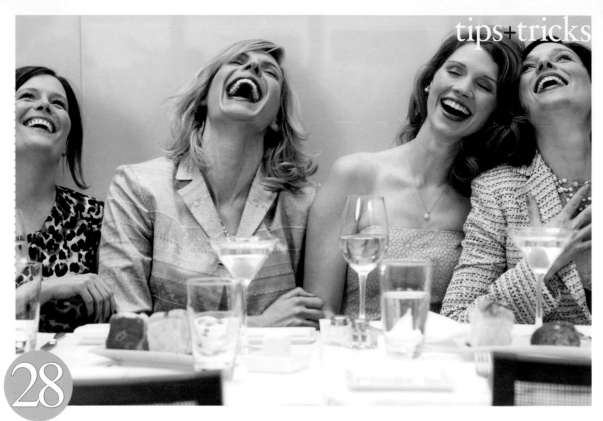

28

my restaurant rules...

01 *Decide what kind of meal you feel like eating before looking at the menu. Don't let yourself get confused with the abundant options.*

02 *Skip the complimentary bread - just say 'no thanks' so that you're not tempted if it's sitting in front of you.*

03 *Avoid the words fried, battered and crumbed - instead go for the steamed, grilled, oven-baked and seared menu options.*

04 *Sip on water throughout the meal, and if you like wine, then order a glass each instead of sharing a bottle between two.*

05 *Why not order an entree as your main? Restaurants tend to overfill the plate, so entree size meals are usually more than enough.*

06 *Share an occasional dessert instead of ordering your own.*

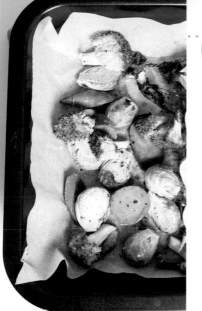

29

veg out

Vegetables, particularly green leafy and cruciferous varieties, are nature's gift to our health. Each type is created differently but perfectly to offer our bodies an abundance of vitamins, minerals and nutrients - all with very little calories. Reduce your waistline and increase the alkalinity of your blood by enjoying as many fresh vegetables as possible.

> **Eat the rainbow** The more colorful vegetables on your plate, the more different nutrients you're getting inside your body.

> **Greens, glorious greens!** You don't have to limit your intake of broccoli, spinach, kale, celery, cucumbers, watercress, rocket, bok choy and lettuces, as they are the purest and simplest detoxing foods on earth.

> **Dip in** Pair veggie sticks and cherry tomatoes with bean dip or guacamole for a balanced and satisfying snack.

> **Who says you can't have veg for breakfast?** Sautéed kale, steamed broccoli, oven-baked beetroot hash browns and grilled zucchini fritters can all be pre-prepared and go well with an egg.

> **Super salads** Excite your salads by adding special touches like freshly sliced mango, pomegranate seeds, grilled figs or honey-candied walnuts.

30 *keep up the challenge!*

It's important to understand WHAT is posing the challenge in every exercise you do. In just about all of the exercises in this 30-day program, it's a combination of your body weight and gravity.
By knowing what's applying the stress or load to an exercise, you'll be able to modify it yourself. That way if you're finding an exercise a little hard, you can change it. If it's too easy you can also change it. To change the effect of gravity you generally need to change the position of your body. For example, by taking a bridge from forearms on the ground to forearms on a table, you're reducing the effect of gravity pushing your hips to the ground. Alternatively you could go from your toes to your knees so that you're not having to hold as much weight off the ground. Any exercise can be modified like this to make it the most suitable version for you.

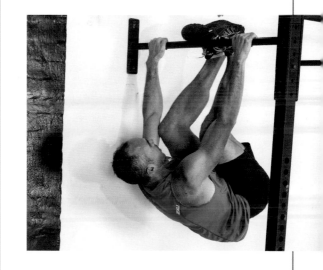

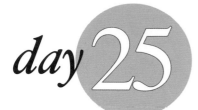

day 25

V holds

MOVEMENT TYPE
BRACE

why?
This is a toughie. It's supine, so nicely balances your recent other body positions. Like the V sit ups, its challenge lies in controlling both your upper and lower body simultaneously.

how?
Sit on the ground with your knees at 90 degrees. Lean back slightly with your torso and lift both feet a few inches off the ground. Hold this position. If by chance you're finding this comfortable you can up the ante by extending your legs and lowering your torso further back.

your record

DATE				
level reached				

The unwanted tendency for this exercise is to hunch your back. You may need to sit more upright to avoid this. Think about pinching your shoulder blades together, opening up your chest, lifting up through your spine and keeping your eyes fixed on a spot above the horizon.

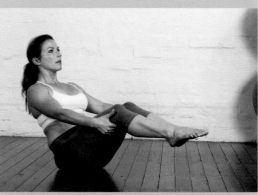

easier version

V holds too hard? Place your fingertips lightly on your hamstrings to provide some stability and support or keep your feet on the ground and lean your torso back. Alternatively, perform the same move as above but place your hands on the ground just behind your backside (fingers facing you) to provide assistance.

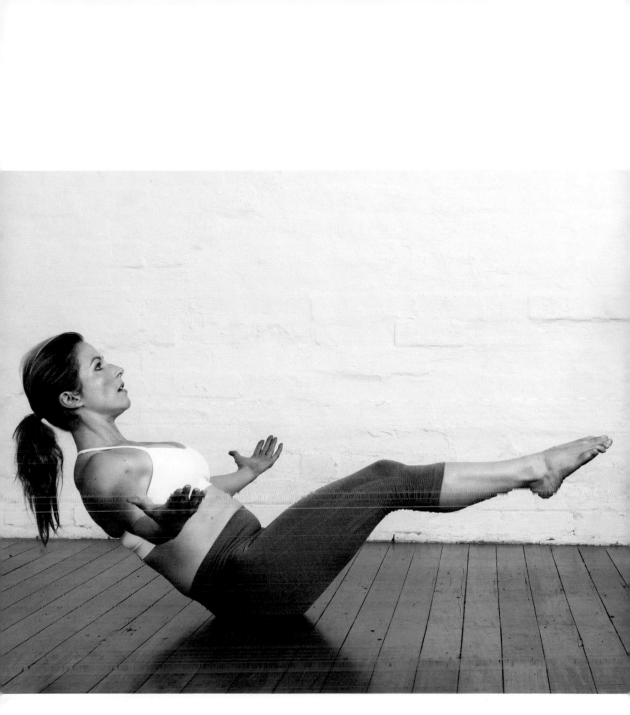

THE CHALLENGE LIES IN
CONTROLLING BOTH YOUR
UPPER AND LOWER BODY
SIMULTANEOUSLY.

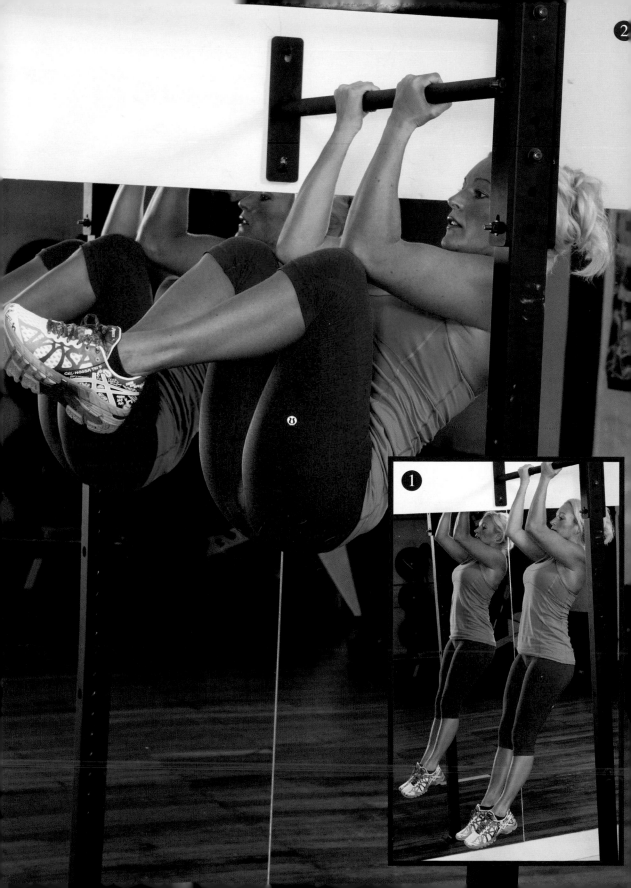

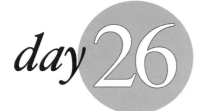
hang elbow to knee

MOVEMENT TYPE
SPINAL FLEXION

targets	BLACK	BLUE	RED
	100	60	20

why?
Simply, it's one of the best exercises to hit your six-pack muscles on the planet. It may take a while and some practise to be able to get your knees all the way up to your elbows but don't worry, just do your best and you'll reap the benefits.

how?
You'll need an overhead horizontal bar for this one. Take a relatively close grip and have palms facing behind you and elbows pointing forward. The move has you taking your feet off the ground then drawing your knees up until they simultaneously touch your elbows. You'll crunch and squeeze through your abs to achieve this. Lower your legs to vertical then repeat. Put your feet back on the ground only if you need to.

Unlike our friends at Crossfit, I don't recommend you use swinging to help get your knees up. When it comes to abs and core it's control that wins hands down. Try to go slow on the down phase (about 3 seconds) and really tuck your tailbone under as you lift up to get your abs working most effectively.

your record

DATE				
level reached				

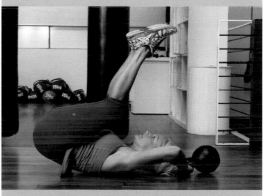

easier version

hang elbow to knee too hard?
Instead of hanging off a bar, lie on your back and grab an anchor point like the underside of a couch or bed. Have your elbows pointing up to the roof. Keeping a firm hold lift your tailbone off the ground and try to touch knees to elbows.

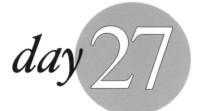
swiss ball jack knives

MOVEMENT TYPE
BRACE

targets

	BLACK	BLUE	RED
	150	100	50

why?

Day by day we have been progressing to harder and more challenging versions of each of our core and abs moves. When it comes to the prone moves we've done supermans, planks, core climbers, arm extensions, brazilians, nose touches, mountain jumpers, supermans and now this one. Each building on the last and challenging your core a little bit more.

how?

Start with the ball behind you and place one shin on top. Now place both your hands on the ground out in front. Stabilising through your leg on the ball, lift the other leg and also place it on the ball. Pause and make sure your body is completely straight with your core engaged to counteract a downward sag of your hips and stomach. Now roll the ball in, bringing your knees towards your chest in a tuck, pause, then roll the ball back until your body is once again long, straight and stable.

When you feel more confident, start with the ball further down your shins then, harder still, try it with your feet on the ball. The gold standard is with only your toes on the ball.

your record

DATE				
level reached				

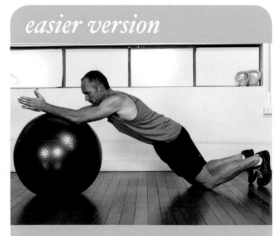

easier version

SB Jack Knives too hard? Still using the ball, kneel in front of it. With the ball about 30cm away, place both forearms on top of the ball in a karate-chop fashion. Brace your core then roll the ball away. Go as far as you can without losing your strong shape. Pause, roll back in and go again.

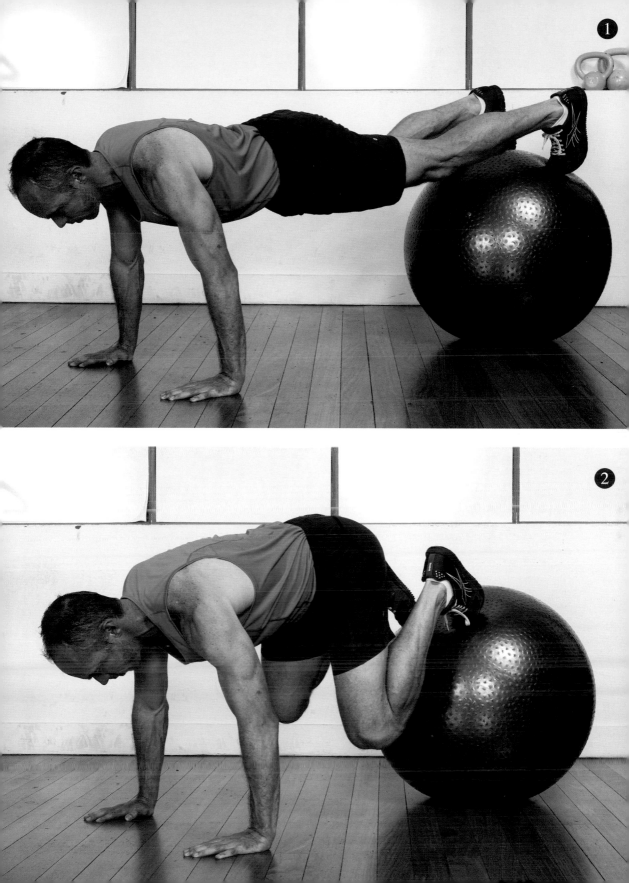

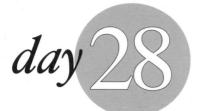

day 28

side bridge transitions

MOVEMENT TYPE
BRACE

targets

	BLACK	BLUE	RED
	75	50	25

why?
Not only will this get your obliques pumping, it'll also a full-body move. Your arms and shoulders will be working hard, as will your lower body.

how?
Lie on your left hand side with your elbow directly under your shoulder. Your body should be perfectly straight, with your left forearm running perpendicular to your torso. Raise your hips off the ground so that you are in a side bridge position. Hold this position for a few seconds and feel the strain in your left obliques. Now roll your right shoulder forward and place your right forearm directly beside your left on the ground. Your torso is now facing the ground, like a bridge. Now raise your left arm and transition into a right arm side bridge position. Try to perform this transition in a controlled yet flowing fashion. That's one rep.

If you rush these your technique will get sloppy. Focus on keeping your hips up, your head in posture and your long, strong alignment throughout.

your record

DATE				
level reached				

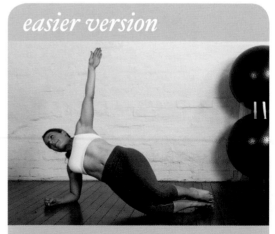

easier version

side bridge transitions too hard?
Try this on your knees until you're ready for the difficult toe version.

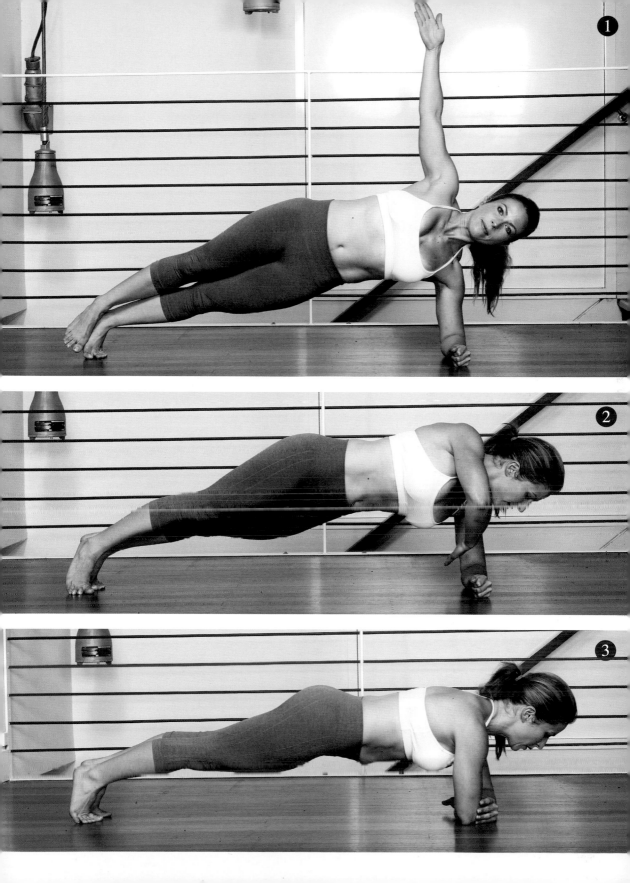

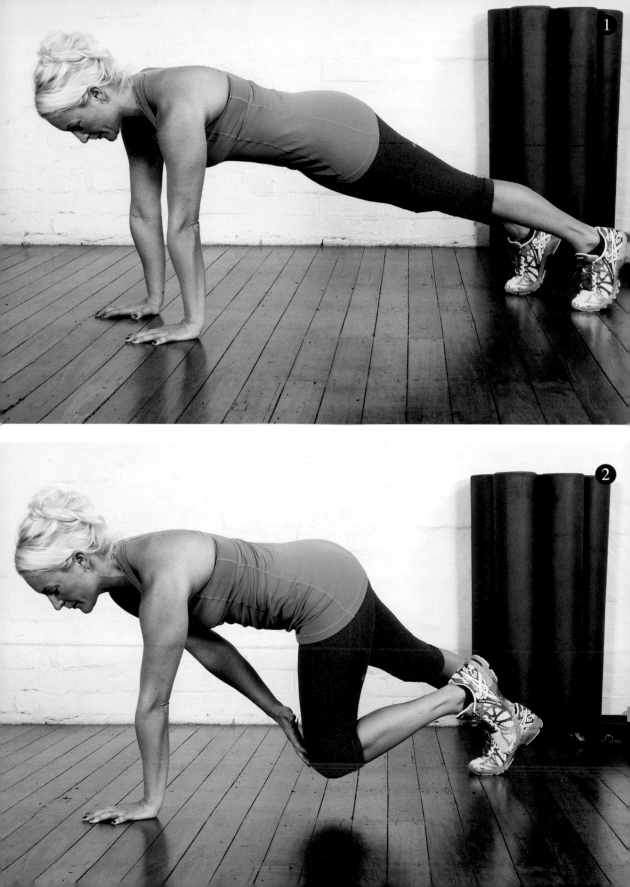

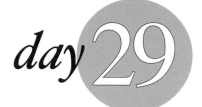

prone hand to knee

MOVEMENT TYPE
BRACE TWIST

why?

This is top of the pops when it comes to core moves. If you can master this, you're the master.

how?

Assume a push-up position with your feet wide apart. Brace your core and hold your body straight. Raise your right arm and left leg off the ground. Touch your hand to your knee. It's easier said than done but do everything you can to avoid your torso twisting and turning. The more your torso remains still the better your core is stabilising you. Alternate arms and legs and do the desired reps. For best results do this move super slow. 3-4 seconds per rep is ideal.

your record

DATE				
level reached				

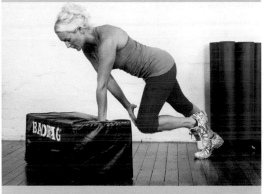

easier version

prone hand to knee too hard?
Try the same general move but rather than having your hands on the ground have them on a raised surface like a bench or ledge.

Yes, it's not that hard to touch your hand to your knee in a prone position but do it with a still torso is another thing altogether. You'll need your TVA and obliques super strong to be able to pull this one off.

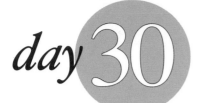

hang toes to bar

MOVEMENT TYPE
SPINAL FLEXION

targets

	BLACK	BLUE	RED
	50	35	20

why?

This exercise is a worthy recipient of the day thirty mantle. It's super tough, but attainable. If you can't manage the black level this time around why not set it as a goal for the future? I guarantee once you can manage it your abs will be in amazing shape.

how?

This is our second move amongst the last 5 to involve a horizontal chin-up type bar. Grasp the bar in an overhand grip with hands shoulder-width apart. Lift your feet off the ground and you're ready to go. Using your new found incredible abdominal strength, lift your legs up and sweep them all the way up until you simultaneously touch both sets of toes to the bar. Slowly lower over about three seconds, pause at vertical (feet should remain off the ground) then go again. Try to minimise any swinging at the bottom.

If your grip strength is what's stopping you progressing with this exercise you may want to invest in some hanging abs straps. These allow you to get all the same abs benefits but mean your not hanging on for dear life.

your record

DATE				
level reached				

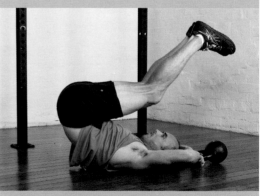

easier version

Hang toes to bar too hard? There are a few options for you here. First do exactly the same move but go to horizontal (half way up) instead of the bar. Still too hard or no bar? Lie on your back, hands grasped to the bottom of a couch (or similar) then raise your feet up and touch your toes to somewhere near your hands. It's a horizontal version of the hanging move.

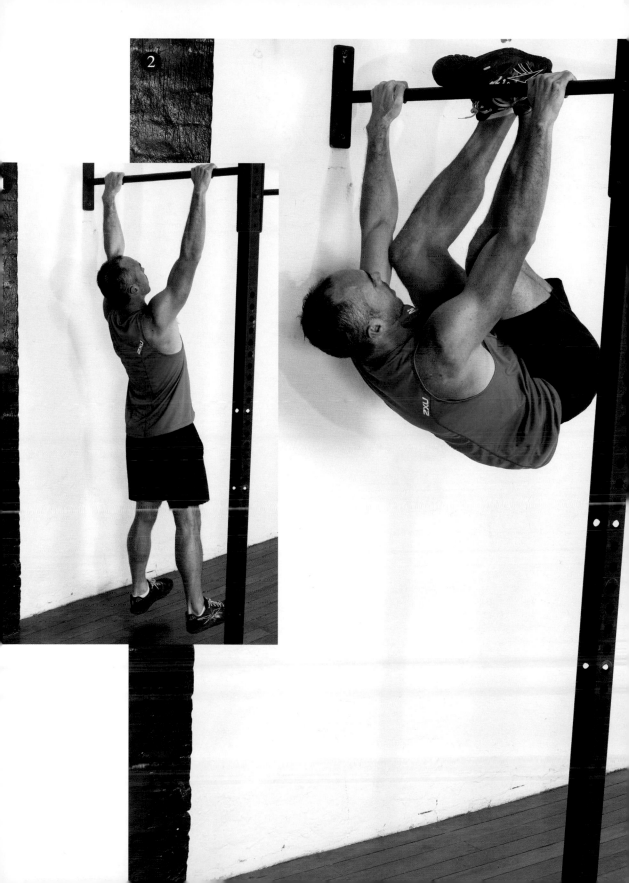

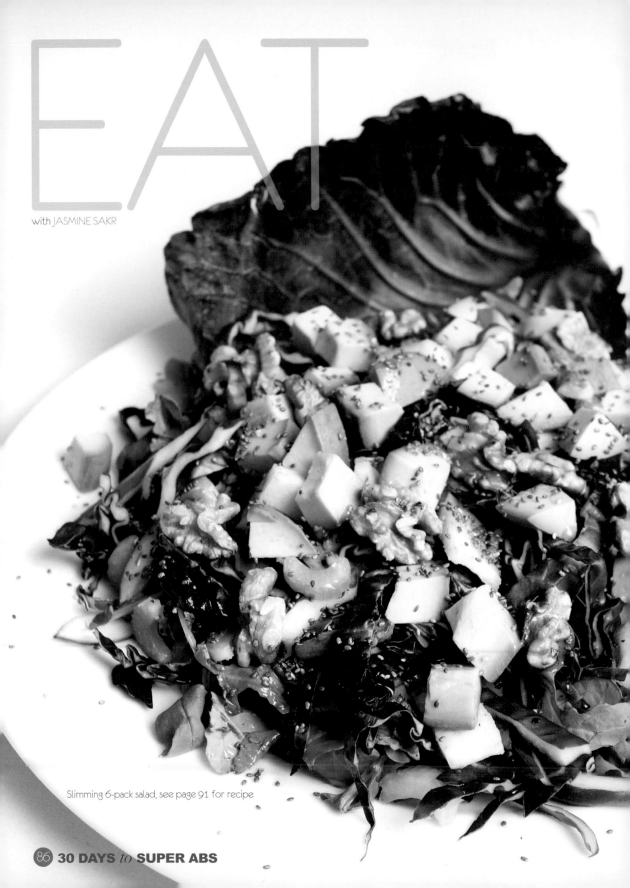

EAT

with JASMINE SAKR

Slimming 6-pack salad, see page 91 for recipe

the new kitchen staples

There are literally thousands of products to choose from every time you visit the supermarket. How much time have you spent comparing nutritional information panels on food packets? Grocery shopping doesn't have to be so complicated. If you stock up on healthy kitchen staples, you'll save money, time and effort.

We've put together a list of versatile basics that should form the foundation of your food shopping, every week. You'll never be short of last minute meals or nutritious snacks with these great ingredients on hand. Simply choose 3 grocery items from every section each week. Experiment and start to utilise these star ingredients in your cooking.

ANIMAL PROTEIN
(preferably organic & free range)
> Eggs
> Milk
> Cheese – opt for white cheese rather than yellow, like haloumi and fetta
> Yoghurt – Greek or plain, not flavoured
> Chicken – breast or thigh is most versatile
> Smoked or fresh salmon/ocean trout
> Fresh, unprocessed seafood to your liking, such as fish fillets and prawns
> Lean red meat, if desired

VEGETABLES AND FRUITS
(preferably local, seasonal produce)
> Green vegetables (as many as you like): broccoli, spinach, kale, celery, cucumbers, watercress, rocket, bok choy and lettuces
> Naturally sweet veggies: tomatoes, carrots, sweet potatoes, pumpkin, corn and peas
> Apples, pears, bananas, stone fruits, melon and fresh or frozen berries as well as avocado
> Garlic, onions, ginger, lemons and fresh herbs, like coriander

GRAINS
> Brown rice – any size grain
> Whole rolled oats
> Quinoa – any colour

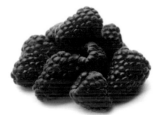

SWEETENERS
> Raw honey, rice malt syrup
> Maple syrup – not maple flavoured
> Naturally dried (unsulphured) fruits: sultanas, raisins, apricots, dates
> ground cinnamon
> unrefined green stevia

BEVERAGES
> Spring water, if desired
> Teas – peppermint, chamomile, jasmine, green, dandelion root (try as a coffee substitute)
> Coconut water

PLANT PROTEIN
> Lentils – any colour
> Chickpeas – canned or dried
> Canned bean mix
> Tofu
> Roasted or raw unsalted nuts – cashews, almonds (can be tamari), walnuts, Brazil
> Seeds – linseeds, sunflower, pepita, chia

CONDIMENTS
> Quality extra virgin olive oil
> Tamari soy sauce
> Sea salt
> Black pepper
> Balsamic vinegar
> Apple cider vinegar
> Dried herbs and spices
> Coconut – milk, oil, shredded

You'll never be short of last-minute meals or nutritious snacks with these great ingredients on hand.

breakfast

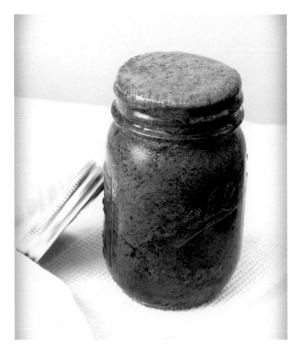

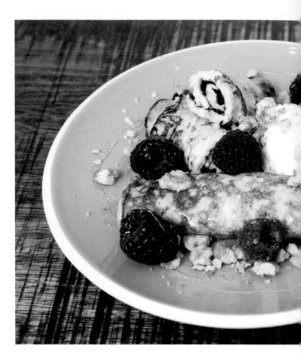

super spirulina protein smoothie

serves 1

WHAT YOU NEED
1 cup (250ml) milk of choice
(organic full cream, unsweetened oat or almond)
2 tbsp Greek yoghurt
½ banana
½ cup ice
¼ cup blueberries
½ tsp spirulina

HOW TO MAKE IT
Blend all ingredients together and enjoy.

For an extra protein hit add a tablespoon of non-artifical protein powder. For extra fibre add ground linseeds (flaxseed). Use frozen berries if fresh are too expensive or not in season.

easy flour-free pancakes

serves 1

WHAT YOU NEED
1 ripe banana, mashed
2 eggs
½ tsp cinnamon
½ tsp vanilla

HOW TO MAKE IT
Whisk all ingredients together in a mixing bowl. In a heated frypan, melt some coconut oil, then cook pancakes, being careful not to let them burn. Note - they will be done very quickly, only about 30 seconds on each side. Get them while they're hot!

Try serving with ricotta, berries and raw honey; pecan nuts and pure maple syrup or shredded coconut and walnuts.

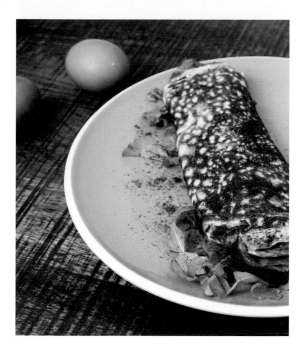

bread-free breakfast wrap

serves 1

WHAT YOU NEED
2 slices smoked salmon
2 eggs
handful rocket/arugula
1 tomato, sliced
cayenne pepper to season

HOW TO MAKE IT
1. Whisk eggs and cayenne pepper in a bowl, then pour into a hot frypan and cook as omelette. Slide omelette onto serving plate.
2. Assemble smoked salmon, rocket and tomato in the middle of the omelette, then roll into a wrap. Enjoy as a protein-rich substitute to sandwich wraps.

Why not add avocado for extra creaminess or substitute smoked salmon for poached chicken or nitrate-free ham. Have fun with different seasonings, spices and fresh herbs!

snack time

bliss balls

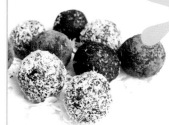

For an easy snack try apple slices with nut butter (use organic, unwaxed apples where possible) or a boiled egg and glass of coconut water.

makes 16-24 balls

WHAT YOU NEED
1 cup medjool dates (soaked)
1 cup ground cashews
½ cup almond meal
¼ cup linseeds (ground)
¼ cup sesame seeds
½ cup dessicated coconut
½ cup raw cocoa powder
1 tsp coconut oil

HOW TO MAKE IT
Combine all ingredients in a food processor until a moist dough is formed. Roll into balls and coat with chia seeds, raw cocoa powder or dessicated coconut. Refrigerate until firm. Store in the refrigerator for freshness.

nutty muesli bars

WHAT YOU NEED
2 mashed ripe bananas
2 tbsp raw organic honey
1 tbsp coconut oil
2 cups whole rolled oats or rolled spelt
1 cup crushed walnuts
½ cup chia seeds
½ cup shredded coconut
1 tbsp pepita seeds
1 tbsp ground cinnamon

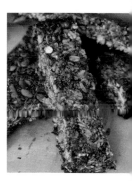

HOW TO MAKE IT
Combine bananas, raw organic honey and coconut oil. Add oats, walnuts, chia seeds, coconut, pepita seeds and cinnamon, combining well. Pour into a lined tin and bake in preheated 180°C/350°F oven for 25 minutes or until golden. Once cooled, cut into bars and store in airtight container. Makes 12.

lunch

Add a dollop of unsweetened Greek yoghurt, substitute beef for chicken or prawns or use whichever vegetable toppings you like, e.g. mushrooms, corn, carrots.

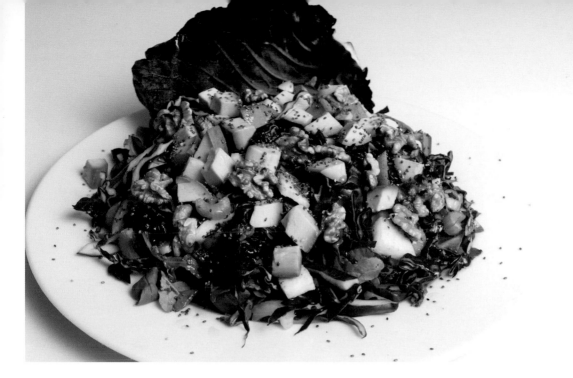

mexican baked sweet potato

serves 2

WHAT YOU NEED
2 large sweet potatoes
1 diced onion
2 garlic cloves, crushed
1 tsp cumin
1 tsp paprika
250g/9 oz beef
2 tomatoes, diced
1 cup rocket/arugula leaves
½ avocado, sliced
½ red capsicum/pepper, sliced
coriander/cilantro and lime to garnish

HOW TO MAKE IT

1. In a 180°C/350°F oven, bake whole sweet potatoes for approx 30 minutes or until skin is slightly blistered and flesh is softened - no wrapping needed, just straight onto a tray.

2. Meanwhile, in a hot frypan, brown onion and garlic together. Mix in cumin and paprika. Add beef and cook until just brown.

3. Finally add diced tomatoes and simmer on low heat for 10 minutes. Take beef mixture off heat once thickened.

4. To assemble, slice sweet potatoes lengthways, and push flesh into the skin with the back of a spoon. Fill pocket with beef, and then top with rocket, avocado, red capsicum. Garnish with a sprinkling of fresh

slimming 6-pack salad

serves 2

WHAT YOU NEED
½ purple/red cabbage
1 cup rocket/arugula leaves
2 stalks celery, sliced
1 pear, cubed
½ avocado, sliced
½ cup toasted walnuts
1 tbsp chia seeds
Dressing
2 tbsp raw honey
2 tbsp olive oil
juice of 1 lemon

HOW TO MAKE IT

1. In a jar, combine honey, olive oil and lemon juice and shake until dressing is formed.

2. In a salad bowl, combine all other ingredients then toss dressing through until well coated.

Rich in essential good fats and fibre!

dinner

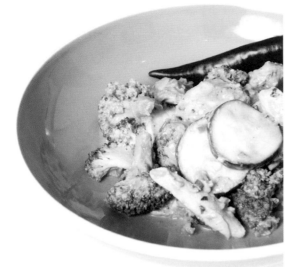

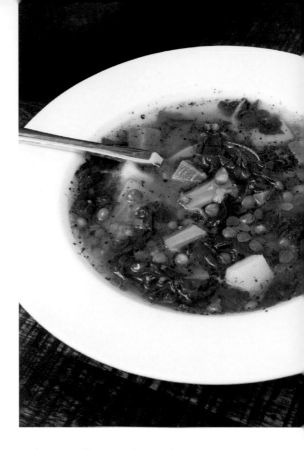

clean, lean chicken satay

serves 4

WHAT YOU NEED

1 tbsp coconut oil
4 spring onions/scallions, chopped
3 organic chicken breasts
green veggies such as sliced zucchini/courgette
and broccoli florets
3 garlic cloves, crushed
1 tsp cumin
1 tsp coriander powder
3 tbsp quality sugar-free crunchy peanut butter
(Peanut allergy? Try another nut butter).
1 tsp chilli, crushed
juice of lemon
brown rice to serve

HOW TO MAKE IT

1. Get your brown rice going as that takes around 25 minutes to cook.
2. Heat 1 tbsp coconut oil in a pan and brown the spring onions. Cut chicken into strips and add to the pan until just cooked.
3. Toss in the broccoli and zucchini (or your choice). Reduce heat, add lid and steam for a few minutes.
4. Transfer to covered dish so chicken and vegetables continue to steam.
5. Heat 1 tbsp coconut oil in the empty pan. Add garlic, spices and peanut butter and stir until combined. Add lemon juice and chilli then add water slowly until desired consistency reached. Return chicken and vegetables to pan and simmer for few minutes. Serve with brown rice.

detoxifying lentil + silverbeet

serves 4

WHAT YOU NEED

1 cup lentils (sorted & rinsed with cold water)
2 potatoes, cubed
8 cups (2L) water
4 cups thinly chopped silverbeet
1 cup freshly squeezed lemon juice
2 or 3 garlic cloves, crushed
1/4 cup sumac
1/2 cup (125ml) olive oil
Salt to taste

HOW TO MAKE IT

1. Boil lentils on medium heat for 5 minutes.
2. Add potatoes and boil together for another 5 minutes.
3. Add water and silverbeet, lower heat and cook for about 30 minutes, stirring occasionally.
4. Mix lemon juice, garlic, sumac, olive oil and salt, add to soup and simmer for a few minutes.
5. Taste and adjust seasoning with garlic, sumac, salt and lemon juice.

broccoli, leek and chilli soup

WHAT YOU NEED
1 leek, chopped
coconut oil
1 tsp chilli flakes
2 chopped broccoli heads
4 cups (1L) MSG-free vegetable stock

HOW TO MAKE IT
1. Saute leek in coconut oil, add chilli flakes, broccoli and stock.
2. Simmer for 20 minutes then blitz everything with a hand held or counter top blender.
3. For added protein, serve with a handful of chickpeas, a dollop of natural yoghurt, crushed walnuts or parmesan cheese.

Make a big batch of this delicious soup and keep refrigerated or frozen in portions for easy lunches and dinners.

index

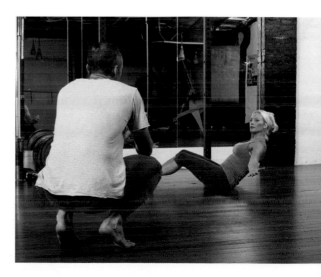

continue your fitness journey...

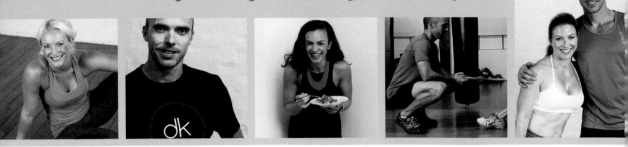

If my 30 Days to Super Abs book has whet your appetite for super smart training, visit our website at www.damienkelly.com.au

acknowledgements

Putting together a book like this is a huge team effort. Thanks firstly to supermodel Sonie for your über good looks and envious core strength. To photographer Rod Stewart, you are a true professional and a true gentleman. Shooting two books in a weekend, let alone with such quality pictures, would have been an impossible task with anyone else. To wonder nutritionist Jasmine. This book desperately needed a nutrition component and I'm so glad we could work together on this exciting project. Your flair for healthy and delicious cooking is second to none. To model number two, my partner in crime Melinda. Not only do I thank you for the use of your amazing 'mother-of -two' bod for these pages but your countless hours to put this book together visually. Your design skills once again allow my workouts to jump off the page into our reader's loungerooms. We met putting together magazines - who would have thought we'd eventually be making books together! And finally, to publisher Michael Wilkinson - thank you again for your boundless faith, enthusiasm and for the opportunity to do our second book together.

Lastly, thank YOU for reading this book and hopefully by now finishing your first dk inspired 30 Days to Super Abs Challenge. You inspire me and everyone around you.

get in touch
Damien Kelly Fitness Studio
118 Bronte Road Bondi Junction 2022
Sydney, Australia. +61 2 8086 2483
damien@damienkelly.com.au

damien kelly *fitness*